The FPPE Toolbox

Field-Tested Documents for Credentialing, Competency, and Compliance

Carol S. Cairns, CPMSM, CPCS
Sally J. Pelletier, CPMSM, CPCS
Donna K. Goestenkors, CPMSM

The FPPE Toolbox: Field-tested Documents for Credentialing, Competency, and Compliance is published by HCPro, Inc.

Copyright © 2008 HCPro, Inc.

ISBN 978-1-60146-157-5

HCPro, Inc., provides information resources for the healthcare industry.

HCPro, Inc., is not affiliated in any way with The Joint Commission, which owns the JCAHO and Joint Commission trademarks.

Carol S. Cairns, CPMSM, CPCS, Author
Sally J. Pelletier, CPMSM, CPCS, Author
Donna K. Goestenkors, CPMSM, Author
Emily Berry, Editor
Maureen Coler, Executive Editor
Bob Croce, Group Publisher
Brian Babineau, Layout Artist

Leah Tracosas, Copyeditor
Lauren Rubenzahl, Proofreader
Jackie Diehl Singer, Graphic Artist
Darren Kelly, Books Production Supervisor
Susan Darbyshire, Art Director
Jean St. Pierre, Director of Operations

Advice given is general. Readers should consult professional counsel for specific legal, ethical, or clinical questions.

Arrangements can be made for quantity discounts. For more information, contact:

HCPro, Inc.
P.O. Box 1168
Marblehead, MA 01945
Telephone: 800/650-6787 or 781/639-1872
Fax: 781/639-2982
E-mail: *customerservice@hcpro.com*

Visit HCPro at its World Wide Web sites:
www.hcpro.com and **www.hcmarketplace.com**

Contents

About the authors...vi

Acknowledgments ix

Introduction x

Editor's note on the text..xiii

Chapter 1: CareLink of Jackson, Jackson, MI 1

Figure 1.1: Focused professional practice evaluation policy/procedure 3

Figure 1.2: Medical staff quality management: Professional practice evaluation
for medical staff assessment 6

Figure 1.3: Medical staff quality management: Professional
practice evaluation for administration/nursing assessment..8

Figure 1.4: Medical staff proctoring policy/procedure.. 10

Figure 1.5: Proctoring evaluation form 13

Figure 1.6: Proctoring summary report... 15

Figure 1.7: Proctor letter 17

Figure 1.8: Letter for the proctored practitioner 18

Chapter 2: Mercy Medical Center, Nampa, ID 19

Figure 2.1: Focused professional practice evaluation policy and procedure 20

Figure 2.2: Emergency department proctor report... 25

Figure 2.3: Surgical proctor report... 27

Figure 2.4: Performance feedback process for mid-level practitioners...................................... 29

Figure 2.5: Performance feedback algorithm for mid-level practitioners 31

Figure 2.6: Nurse midwife proctor report 32

Figure 2.7: Proctoring by department... 34

Chapter 3: MeritCare Health System, Fargo, ND 37

Figure 3.1: Focused professional practice evaluations 38

Figure 3.2: Departmental policy on focused professional practice evaluations 47

Figure 3.3: Prospective proctoring: Cognitive diagnostic/Medical evaluation form.................... 49

Figure 3.4: Concurrent proctoring: Cognitive diagnostic/medical evaluation form.................... 51

Figure 3.5: Prospective proctoring procedural/surgical evaluation form................................... 53

Figure 3.6: Concurrent proctoring: Procedural/surgical evaluation form................................... 55

Figure 3.7: Retrospective proctoring: Case rating form 57

Figure 3.8: Ongoing physician feedback policy 59

Figure 3.9: Anesthesia: Focused professional physician evaluation plan 62

Figure 3.10: Anesthesia: Focused professional physician evaluation plan for CRNA 63

Figure 3.11: Critical care medicine: Proctoring policy 65

Figure 3.12: Emergency: Focused professional physician evaluation plan............................... 66

Figure 3.13: Pediactrics: Focused professional physician evaluation plan 67

Figure 3.14: Psychiatry: Focused professional physician evaluation plan............................... 69

Figure 3.15: Urology: Focused professional physician evaluation plan 71

Chapter 4: St. John's Health System, Springfield, MO 73

Figure 4.1 Monitoring and peer review policy 74

Figure 4.2 Chart review for peer review/case review referrals.................................... 77

Figure 4.3 Proctoring program for practitioners 79

Figure 4.4 Proctoring program algorithm 84

Figure 4.5 Proctoring letter and checklist 85

Figure 4.6 Procedure log to document proctored cases or privilege maintenance 87

Editor's note 88

Figure 4.7 Cardiovascular proctor checklist... 89

Figure 4.8 Cardiovascular and thoracic surgery proctor checklist 91

Figure 4.9 Emergency medicine proctor checklist 92

Figure 4.10 Family medicine/sports medicine proctor checklist 93

Figure 4.11 Gastroenterology proctor checklist 96

Figure 4.12 Neurological surgery proctor checklist... 97

Figure 4.13 Urology proctor checklist 99

Chapter 5: XYZ Medical Center **101**

Figure 5.1 Medicine service professional practice evaluation 102

Figure 5.2 Dental service professional practice evaluation 104

Chapter 6: Additional FPPE documents **107**

Figure 6.1 Focused professional practice evaluation process... 107

Figure 6.2: Guide to drafting a focused professional practice evaluation policy 110

Figure 6.3: Sample focused professional practice evaluation plan

　　　　for a newly trained and board-certified cardiologist ....

Figure 6.4: Sample focused professional practice evaluation plan for a nurse midwife 112

Follow these simple steps to earn your CE credits 113

Carol S. Cairns, CPMSM, CPCS

Carol S. Cairns has participated in the development of the medical staff services profession for more than 35 years. She is a senior consultant and frequent presenter with The Greeley Company, based in Marblehead, MA, and is the president of PRO-CON, an Illinois consulting firm specializing in credentialing, privileging, medical staff organization operations, and survey preparation. A recognized expert in the field, Cairns presents frequently for healthcare entities as well as at state and national seminars.

Cairns began her career in medical staff services in Joliet, IL, where she coordinated and directed medical staff services for Provena Saint Joseph Medical Center and Silver Cross Hospital. In 1991, Cairns became clinical faculty for The Joint Commission by collaboratively developing an educational program entitled "Credentialing and Privileging Medical Staff and Allied Health Professionals." She served as clinical faculty for this program from 1991 to 2000. For The Joint Commission, Cairns coauthored *The Medical Staff Handbook: A Guide to Joint Commission Standards*, which focuses on medical staff credentialing and privileging standards, and authored *The LIP's Guide to Credentials Review and Privileging*.

In addition, Cairns has been a faculty member with the National Association Medical Staff Services (NAMSS) since 1990. She has presented at numerous state and national seminars on subjects such as basic and advanced credentialing and privileging, the Centers for Medicare & Medicaid Services' *Conditions of Participation*, The Joint Commission standards and survey preparation, National Committee on Quality Assurance (NCQA) standards, American Osteopathic Association Healthcare Facilities Accreditation Program Standards, AHP credentialing, core privileging, risk management, and meeting management and documentation. In 1995, Cairns coauthored the NAMSS educational program for certification of provider credentialing specialists (CPCS), for which she also currently serves as faculty.

In 1996, NCQA appointed Cairns as a surveyor in its certification program for credentials verification organizations (CVO). She surveyed CVOs for the NCQA and was a clinical faculty member for the NCQA on credentialing and CVO certification until 2006. In 2003, Cairns provided input to the American Osteopathic Association 2004 Healthcare Facilities Accreditation Program relative to the medical staff and allied health professionals credentialing and privileging standards.

In 2005, the Illinois State Association Medical Staff Services recognized Cairns by presenting her with a Distinguished Member award. To date, she is the only recipient.

Other HCPro, Inc., books authored or coauthored by Cairns include *Verify and Comply: A Quick Reference Guide to The Joint Commission and NCQA Standards for Credentialing*; *A Guide to AHP Credentialing: Challenges and Opportunities to Credentialing Allied Health Professionals*; *Core Privileges for Physicians: A Practical Approach to Development and Implementation, Fourth Edition*; and *Core Privileges for AHPs: A Practical Approach to Development and Implementing Criteria-Based Privileges.*

Sally J. Pelletier, CPMSM, CPCS

Sally J. Pelletier, serves as a senior consultant for The Greeley Company. She brings more than 15 years of credentialing and privileging experience to her work with medical staff leaders and medical service professionals across the nation. Pelletier advises in the areas of criteria-based core privileging, MSO assessments, and medical staff services management.

In 2004, she began consulting with The Greeley Company. Pelletier also writes a biweekly e-newsletter column for HCPro's *Credentialing and Privileging Advisor*. In addition, she is a contributing editor to the **Briefings on Credentialing** newsletter and has coauthored *Converting to Core Privileging* and *Core Privileges for Physicians, Fourth Edition,* all of which are published by HCPro.

Pelletier presents at state and national seminars on such topics as basic and advanced credentialing and privileging, allied health practitioners, core privileging, background checks, and physician aging.

She is currently secretary for NAMSS. Her other leadership roles for NAMSS have included chair of the Governance, Management and Manpower Committee; chair of the Bylaws Committee; chair of the Credentialing Elements Task Force; and member of the Credentialing Consensus Alliance. In addition, she served as president of the New Hampshire Association Medical Staff Services.

Prior to joining The Greeley Company, Pelletier was a consultant for SJP Pro Med Enterprise and medical staff coordinator for The Memorial Hospital in North Conway, NH.

Pelletier is certified by NAMSS as a certified professional medical services manager (CPMSM) and a certified provider credentials specialist (CPCS).

Donna K. Goestenkors, CPMSM

Donna K. Goestenkors, is a consultant with The Greeley Company who specializes in credentialing and privileging. She brings more than 30 years of credentialing and accreditation experience to her work with hospitals, medical staff offices (MSOs), healthcare systems, credentials committees, health plans, medical groups, bylaws committees, and CVOs nationwide.

Goestenkors applies her management experience to helping clients develop solutions to their unique needs and challenges. She has particular expertise in Joint Commission and Centers for Medicare & Medicaid Services (CMS) standards compliance, bylaws, rules and regulations, staffing, credentialing, clinical privileging, MSO operations, budget compliance, and technology improvements. She also advises clients in leadership, office policies, procedures, and best practices.

Goestenkors is a past president of NAMSS. She has authored and contributed to numerous articles and books about medical staff organizational management, including *Medical Staff Services Professionals Take Charge,* published by HCPro Inc. She has also presented many NAMSS and HCPro audioconferences, in addition to doing technical and administrative presentations on Joint Commission standards, federal and state regulations, meeting management, staffing, MSO administration, leadership skills, and credentialing.

Prior to joining The Greeley Company, Goestenkors worked as a manager of medical staff services for BJC HealthCare's Christian Hospital in St. Louis. She was also an outside regulatory advisor and advocate for patient safety in medical services departments in the areas of Joint Commission compliance, rules and regulations, staffing, credentialing, clinical privileging, leadership, and office policies, procedures, and practices. She has also served as an expert witness in litigation cases.

Goestenkors holds an associate's degree in medical services' with concentrations in anatomy, pharmacology, physiology, and medical terminology. She has certified professional medical services management (CPMSM) certification from NAMSS and is a member in good standing. She also is actively pursuing certified provider in healthcare quality (CPHQ) certification from the National Association of Healthcare Quality.

Acknowledgments

Today's practitioners are expected to prove their competency in greater detail than ever before. This brings tremendous benefits for patients. It also challenges medical staff leaders and medical staff professionals, as well as quality managment personnel, to develop policies and practices that help organizations and practitioners meet their obligation to provide evidence of demonstrated current competency. While all of those groups must work on this process together it is essential for medical staff leaders to own their competency evaluations by supplying the criteria and implementing the approved processes.

But where to begin? Competency itself is a complex and subjective idea. Even the definition lacks a straightforward answer. Merriam-Webster's Collegiate Dictionary provides four definitions for competence, including, "having the capacity to function or develop in a particular way…"

If you work at a Joint Commission-accredited facility, it is best to begin your competency research by familiarizing yourself with Joint Commission standard MS 4.30, which requires organizations to validate the competency of newly privileged practitioners. This standard provides the framework you'll need to develop your policies and procedures, and we hope that this book will serve as your toolbox to implement the rest. Even if your facility is not Joint Commission accredited, we hope this book will be just as helpful because The Centers for Medicare & Medicaid Services (CMS) Conditions of Participation (COPs), also contain the expectation that there is evidence related to competency for those privileged individuals.

The information included in this book would not have been possible without the generous contributions of MSPs working in the field and evaluating competency in accordance with standard MS 4.30. We especially thank those contributors as their dedication to the medical staff services profession continues to inspire us. Even when things get difficult for MSPs, they can always find solutions! We also offer thanks to our colleagues at The Greeley Company and everyone in the healthcare field.

"All things should be made as simple as possible, but not more so."
–Albert Einstein

Whatever your healthcare leadership role may be—whether you are a member of the medical staff, administration, medical staff services department, quality improvement department, or risk management department—chances are you are surrounded by terms like patient safety, quality care, and risk management. Yet, the approach each of us takes to ensure that our hospitals provide the best possible care for our communities is unique and customized to our organization's culture.

Although it is unlikely that this uniqueness will disappear entirely, there is an increasing number of similarities developing among Joint Commission (formerly JCAHO)–accredited hospitals who create policies based on the organization's evolving standards. In January 2008, Joint Commission standard MS 4.30 went into effect and requires organizations to validate the competency of newly privileged practitioners. Standard MS 4.30 requires the organized medical staff to implement focused professional practice evaluation (FPPE) for all initially requested privileges. It also requires organized medical staffs to define:

- How monitoring will be conducted at their facility

- When the monitoring will take place

- How a practitioner's professional performance will be evaluated during that monitoring

FPPE extends the previous requirements of The Joint Commission to conduct focused professional practice evaluation when a "question arises regarding a currently privileged practitioner's ability to provide safe, high quality patient care." The differences between the two uses of FPPE are as follows:

1. The intent of FPPE for the newly-privileged is to confirm competence that has been suggested through the initial credentialing and privileging verification and approval processes

2. The FPPE process related to potential practice concerns determines whether there is an issue related to current clinical competence, practice behavior, or ability to perform a requested procedure

Practitioners are mutually accountable to each other for determining competency at appointment and reappointment, and when setting and following privileging criteria. In concert with leadership, they are responsible for developing and improving the processes for measuring and assessing the competency of licensed independent practitioners and other healthcare professionals credentialed and privileged through the medical staff process.

Measuring Physician Competency: How to Collect, Assess, and Provide Performance Data, Second Edition (HCPro, Inc., 2007) and *Proctoring and Focused Professional Practice Evaluation: Practical Approaches to Verifying Physician Competence (HCPro, Inc., 2006)* were written to meet the needs of organizations and leaders struggling with how to develop and implement effective physician competency measurement systems and feedback reports. These books provide readers with a comprehensive overview of the FPPE process.

The FPPE Toolbox: Field-tested Documents for Credentialing, Competency, and Compliance is the perfect companion to these books. It was developed to provide readers with customizable forms, policies, letters, and other documents to use to comply with The Joint Commission's FPPE requirements.

As healthcare leadership coaches and consultants, we in The Greeley Company have seen our share of forms, policies, and flow charts depicting how hospitals and medical staffs have designed their FPPE programs. We have developed this book to elevate your current understanding of FPPE, assist your organization in complying with standard MS 4.30, and, to some degree, help you to make industry-wide connections to meet your personal quality care goals.

In The Greeley Company, we often talk about the Competency Equation.
Competency = Evidence that you did it recently + Evidence that when you did it, you did it well.

Readers will notice that the way organizations have defined "it" varies. Some are using the actual clinical diagnosis or procedure; some are using the six areas of general competencies as defined by the American Council for Graduate Medical Education and the American Board of Medical

Specialties. There are no rules as to how an organization chooses to define "it." Thus, medical staffs are free to develop systems that work for them.

The tools in this book are designed to be adapted to your organization's own credentialing and privileging practices that also meet our best practice standards. The Greeley Company defines four steps in a best practice credentialing and privileging program:

1. Establish policies and rules

2. Collect and summarize information

3. Evaluate and recommend

4. Review, grant, deny, or approve

The field-tested documents in this book typify those four steps and will help you develop a transparent, meaningful, and easy to understand processes for FPPE management. We hope that your organization will benefit from the diversity and sophistication of this collection of resources provided through the generosity of your peers. If you haven't developed your FPPE program, this resource is definitely a great starting point. If you are looking for ways to strengthen your existing program, this toolbox has the components you need.

As you determine which of the following documents is the best fit for your organization's culture, keep in mind that the goal of FPPE is to confirm the competency of a practitioner to exercise specific clinical privileges. We urge you not simply to copy the pages for your use but instead to truly examine and educate yourself on what criteria and triggers will be used to define your FPPE program, identify your organized medical staff's preferred monitoring type (e.g., chart review, monitoring clinical practice patterns, simulation, proctoring, external peer review, and discussions with other individuals involved in the care of each patient), and determine the best time frame for this monitoring.

What you do as a leader does make a difference. Thank you for leaving a lasting legacy of quality.

Throughout the book, the authors highlighted notable sections of documents and formatted their comments as follows:

> ▶ *These note boxes denote comments that apply universally to the document.*

> These thought bubbles denote comments that apply to specific words or sections within the document. The arrow directs the reader to the area to which the comment is referring.

CareLink of Jackson, Jackson, MI

CareLink of Jackson is a freestanding long-term acute care hospital that specializes in treating patients with complex needs, serious wounds, and surgical complications. Care may also include long and short-term ventilator management. The Joint Commission (formerly JCAHO)–accredited facility provides teaching opportunities for nursing and pharmacy students. It is licensed for 64 beds, has a medical staff of 36 members, and based on patient care need may also grant temporary privileges for subspecialty care. In accordance with CareLink's medical staff bylaws, the medical director is a physician appointed to the active staff by the board and contracted by CareLink. He is a full-time practicing pulmonologist, in addition to:

- Being an ex officio member of all medical staff committees

- Chairing the medical executive committee (MEC)

- Being concerned with medical-administrative, medical-legal, and quality aspects of patient care

- Having the disciplinary powers insofar as the medical staff is concerned

- Being responsible for the proper functioning of medical staff affairs, including reporting any adverse situations to the appropriate chief of the clinical service and the vice president/chief operational officer

Angie Brigham, BA, CPMSM, medical staff coordinator at CareLink of Jackson, says that she started developing the organization's focused professional practice evaluation (FPPE) criteria when The Joint Commission's prepublication standards were released. The resulting forms and procedures were a mix of existing and new documents. Brigham adapted the organization's credentialing evaluations, which were based on the six general competencies, for the FPPE and ongoing professional practice evaluations. The FPPE and proctoring policies were newly created, but both include information found in bylaws and other policies.

When CareLink implemented its new FPPE policies, Brigham first drafted the FPPE and proctoring policies, along with the evaluation forms. Then the chief of internal medicine, medical director, vice president/chief operations officer reviewed these documents. Finally, the FPPE documents were approved by the MEC and governing board.

Brigham says that although CareLink has not yet faced any obstacles to implementing its new FPPE policy, it may need to partner with a nearby hospital, of which all medical staff and AHPs are required to be members, to perform some of the proctoring.

| Figure 1.1 | Focused professional practice evaluation policy/procedure |

Note: *This document outlines the organization's policy overall structure for the FPPE process.*

Purpose: To provide a mechanism for monitoring, evaluating, documenting, and reporting the performance of practitioners granted clinical privileges

Policy: Upon appointment to the medical or allied health staff, each practitioner shall have his or her performance monitored, evaluated, documented, and reported to the medical executive committee (MEC) on an ongoing basis. Focused professional practice evaluations shall be performed and documented for each practitioner without documented current performance at the organization, whenever a question arises regarding a practitioner's ability to provide safe and high quality patient care, or as otherwise indicated within the medical staff bylaws and policies. The medical director or his or her designee shall, at any time, immediately act upon any reported concern regarding a privileged practitioner's clinical practice or competence.

Evaluation

Factors to be considered: The criteria used for evaluation include; but are not limited to:
a. Concurrent review of the practitioner's assessment and treatment of patients
b. Review of invasive and noninvasive clinical procedures performed and their outcomes
c. Blood utilization, medication management, and morbidity and mortality data
d. Requests for tests and procedures, use of consultants, and medical records compliance
e. Other relevant criteria as directed within the bylaws or by the MEC

The evaluation process: Information used for evaluation may be obtained through but is not limited to:
a. Concurrent or targeted medical record review
b. Direct observation
c. Monitoring/proctoring
d. Discussion with other practitioners involved in the care of specific patients
e. Data collected and assessed for the organization's quality improvement indicators
f. Sentinel event data
g. Any applicable peer review data

In this organization, the medical director is a practicing pulmonologist who has both clinical and administrative duties, as explained in the profile at the beginning of the chapter.

Process

Initial privileges: Applies to initial applicants or current members requesting new privileges:
a. Evaluations shall be performed by the medical director, the clinical service chief, or an appointed member of the medical staff and may include direct observation of patient care activities, medical record analysis, or means addressed in medical staff bylaws, article III.B. Evaluations shall

| Figure 1.1 | Focused professional practice evaluation policy/procedure (cont.) |

be submitted to the medical staff office (MSO) at least every six months, with their results being presented to the MEC during its next scheduled meeting. Concerns regarding a practitioner's clinical practice or competence shall be acted upon *immediately.*

The MSO shall provide each evaluator with the approved professional practice evaluation form (attachment A) and a confidential return envelope prior to the end of each six-month evaluation period and as requested. Six-month evaluations are to be submitted to the MSO by the deadline indicated on the evaluation form.

b. Monitoring/proctoring of specific procedures shall be performed as required by the clinical service, or upon request of the medical director or clinical service chief. The medical director or clinical service chief of each involved service shall assign a proctor from the medical staff. If a proctor cannot be chosen from the medical staff due to an obvious or perceived potential conflict of interest, the medical director and vice president (VP)/chief operating officer (COO) shall agree upon a proctor who may or may not be a current member of another organization's medical staff.

The MSO shall provide each proctor with the approved proctoring evaluation form (attachment B) and a confidential return envelope as needed. Extra copies are available in the MSO/library. Evaluations shall be submitted to the MSO within 48 hours of the proctoring. Concerns regarding a practitioner's clinical practice or competence are to be immediately reported to the medical director or clinical service chief.

Due to the nature of the hospital, proctoring may occur at another organization, with the approval of the medical director and VP/COO, if the same circumstances (equipment/supplies/support) are available at this organization for future performance of the specified procedure. Completion and submission of this organization's approved proctoring form is required.

Quality of care issues: It is this organization's policy that quality concerns regarding patient care be addressed as they arise to provide continuous quality patient care and safety and to ensure favorable clinical outcomes. A quality concern regarding any practitioner may be raised by medical or allied health staff, nursing staff, or through the performance improvement process. If a collegial approach to the concern is not effective (see the concurrent quality concerns policy), the concerned party will file a written report with the MSO.

The MEC shall review and act upon situations involving questions of the clinical competence, patient care and treatment, case management, or inappropriate behavior of any practitioner. A targeted chart review is warranted whenever the medical director, chief of a clinical service, or the VP/COO:

  a. Has cause to question the demonstrated clinical competence of any practitioner
  b. Has cause to question the care or treatment of a patient or management of a case by any practitioner
  c. Knows of or has reason to suspect violation by any practitioner of applicable ethical standards of the medical staff bylaws, rules and regulations, policies, corporate bylaws, or the corporate responsibility program or standards of conduct

| Figure 1.1 | Focused professional practice evaluation policy/procedure (cont.) |

Quality of care issues should be reported using an occurrence reporting form, disruptive behavior reporting form, or patient grievance flowsheet. These forms are available on each nursing unit and through the MSO. All reports are processed in accordance with medical staff bylaws and the concurrent quality concerns, medical review, and peer review policies.

Any evaluation referencing peer review or quality concern issues shall be submitted to the MEC during its next meeting; however, the medical director or his or her designee shall, at any time, immediately act upon any reported concern regarding a practitioner's clinical practice or competence.

Temporary privileges: Special requirements of supervision and reporting may be imposed upon any individual granted temporary clinical privileges. Notice of any failure by the individual to comply with such special requirements may result in immediate termination of privileges.

Performance/quality issue resolution

This organization supports the medical staff in addressing all quality of care concerns regarding practitioners through a nonbiased and nonpunitive process by which all provider-related occurrences are reviewed, documented, and appropriate action taken. The medical director and MEC shall perform such oversight, with input from the clinical services.

The medical staff peer review policy established the process by which medical staff quality of care reviews such as peer review and unresolved complaints may be resolved in a nonpunitive atmosphere that promotes education, performance improvement, and favorable clinical outcomes. Circumstances requiring peer review are delineated in the peer review policy.

Through this process, each death, resuscitation, and unanticipated transfer is reviewed to reduce morbidity and mortality and to improve the quality of care. The director of development and organizational excellence, an appointed member of the MEC, reviews each patient death, resuscitation, and unanticipated transfer and performs targeted chart reviews using the approved medical review monitors. All monitors are forwarded to the medical director for final review. Completed medical review monitors are maintained in the affected practitioner's confidential peer review file in the MSO. Medical review monitor data is presented during the quarterly MEC meetings.

Approved:

_____

Medical director   Date

_____

Director of development and organizational excellence   Date

_____

Vice president/Chief operating officer   Date

Source: CareLink of Jackson, Jackson, MI

Figure 1.2	Medical staff quality management: Professional practice evaluation for medical staff assessment

Note: *This document serves as attachment A to the focused professional practice evaluation policy/procedure (Figure 1.1). The medical director conducts this assessment twice per year.*

Indicator	Assessment *Comment on last page.					Data Source(s) In addition to credentialing file review) *Comment on last page.
	Superior	Average	Poor*	Complaints*	Trends*	
Patient Care						
1. Assessment of patients						❏ Interdisciplinary team ❏ Chart review ❏ Observation ❏ Staff verbalization ❏ Peer review/reports* ❏ Comments/survey*
2. Development and implementation of patient management plans						
3. Clinical competence and judgment						
4. Consultant utilization						
5. Communication with patients and families						
6. Patient/family counseling and education						
7. Provision of continuous care and supervision to assigned patients						
Medical knowledge, learning, and improvment						
8. Knowledge of basic and discipline-specific medicine						❏ Interdisciplinary team ❏ Chart review ❏ Observation ❏ Staff verbalization ❏ Peer review/reports* ❏ Comments/survey*
9. Locates, appraises, and understands labs, clinical research, patient demographics, etc., and applies this knowledge effectively						
10. Evaluates his or her patient care practices and makes improvements as needed						
11. Proactive in increasing his or her own knowledge base and in facilitating learning in other healthcare professionals						
Interpersonal and communication skills						
12. Therapeutic and ethical relationship with patients, families, and other members of the healthcare team.						❏ Interdisciplinary team ❏ Chart review ❏ Observation ❏ Staff verbalization ❏ Peer review/reports* ❏ Comments/survey*
13. Effective nonverbal, listening, explanatory, questioning, and writing skills						
14. Timely, appropriate, concise communication that facilitates continuity of care/consistency of treatment plan when assuming care of patients and when handing off to next practitioner						
15. Effective as a member of the interdisciplinary healthcare team						
Professionalism						
16. Responsive, accountable, and committed to patients and the profession						❏ Interdisciplinary team ❏ Chart review ❏ Observation ❏ Staff verbalization ❏ Peer review/reports* ❏ Comments/survey*
17. Demonstrates respect, compassion, and integrity						
18. Ethical principles: provision/withholding of clinical care, patient confidentiality, informed consent, and business practices						
19. Demonstrates sensitivity/responsiveness to patient/coworker's culture, age, gender, and disabilities						
20. Physical/mental ability to safely render care						

Figure 1.2	Medical staff quality management: Professional practice evaluation for medical staff assessment (cont.)

21. **Patient satisfaction**	❑ No comments on file ❑ Comments on file: Positive #_____ Negative #_____* ❑ Complaints* ❑ Trends*

22.	**Utilization management**	Number of unanticipated transfers to acute care:
	Assessment:	❑ Appropriate ❑ Trends* ❑ Referred for CME* ❑ Peer review* ❑ Improvement plans*

23.	**Blood usage**	Transfusion of packed cells ordered:
	Assessment:	❑ Appropriate ❑ Trends* ❑ Referred for CME* ❑ Peer review* ❑ Improvement plans*

24.	**Medication management**	❑ Appropriate ❑ Trends* ❑ Referred for CME* ❑ Peer review* ❑ Improvement plans*

25.	**Morbidity and mortality**	❑ None requiring review Mortalities reviewed: _____ Resuscitations reviewed: _____ Targeted reviews: _____ ❑ No adverse outcomes ❑ Medical management appropriate. No quality issues. Minor adverse outcomes: ___ Major adverse outcomes: ___ Care appropriate: ___ Care inappropriate: ___ Medical management controversial: ___ Medical management inappropriate: ___
	Assessment:	❑ No action ❑ System problems* ❑ Referred for CME* ❑ Peer review* ❑ Improvement plans*

26.	**Medical records**	Delinquent: _____ Deficient history and physical:_____ Summary: _____ Orders:_____
	Assessment:	❑ Appropriate ❑ Trends* ❑ Peer review* ❑ Improvement plans*

27.	**Physician orders for lifesaving treatment** (i.e., do not resuscitate orders) (goal = within first 48 hours)	Completed and on file within first 48 hours of admission:
	Assessment:	❑ No Action Warrented ❑ Trends* ❑ Peer review* ❑ Improvement plans*

Comments: _____

Measurements prepopulated by the medical staff office.

Profile reviewed & assessment completed by: _____

Medical director Date

Profile reviewed & accepted by: _____

Vice president/Chief operating officer Date

In this organization, the medical director is a practicing pulmonologist who has both clinical and administrative duties, as explained in the profile at the beginning of the chapter.

Source: CareLink of Jackson, Jackson, MI

Figure 1.3	Medical staff quality managment: Professional practice evaluation for administration/nursing assesment

> **Note:** *This assessment is performed by the vice president/chief operating officer in conjunction with the nursing clinical manager and other staff as appropriate. It is practitioner-specific and is done twice a year.*

Factor	Evaluation C - Comments on last page			Data Source Check all applicable
Patient care	Yes	No	C	
1. Patient assessments are comprehensive, accurate, and current				
2. Timely development, implementation, and revision of patient management plans				❏ Interdisciplinary team
3. Demonstrated clinical competence and judgment				❏ Chart review ❏ Comments on file
4. Appropriate and timely utilization of consultants				❏ Staff verbalization ❏ Observation
5. Appropriate, compassionate, and effective communication with patients/families				❏ Other
6. Compassionate and audience-specific patient/family counseling and education				
Clinical knowledge, learning, and improvement	Yes	No	C	❏ Interdisciplinary team
7. Demonstrates knowledge of basic and discipline-specific medicine				❏ Chart review ❏ Comments on file
8. Timely ordering, appraisal, and follow-up of diagnostic tests				❏ Staff verbalization
9. Proactive and appropriate when facilitating learning in other health-care professionals				❏ Observation ❏ Other
Interpersonal and communication skills	Yes	No	C	
10. Fosters a therapeutic and ethical relationship with patients/families				
11. Fosters a collegial and ethical relationship with members of the healthcare team				❏ Interdisciplinary team
12. Effective nonverbal, listening, explanatory, and questioning skills				❏ Chart review ❏ Comments on file
13. Timely, appropriate, and concise communication that facilitates continuity of care and consistency of treatment plan when assuming care of patients and when handing off to next practitioner				❏ Staff verbalization ❏ Observation ❏ Other
14. Effective as a member of the interdisciplinary healthcare team				
15. Attends/actively participates in interdisciplinary meetings/discussions as required/requested				

| Figure 1.3 | Medical staff quality managment: Professional practice evaluation for administration/nursing assesment (cont.) |

Professionalism	Yes	No	C	
16. Responsive, accountable, and committed to patients, the hospital, and the healthcare team				❑ Interdisciplinary team
17. Timely response to pages and phone messages from members of the healthcare team				❑ Chart review
18. Demonstrates respect, compassion, and integrity in all interactions				❑ Comments on file
19. Demonstrates ethical principles: provision/withholding of clinical care, confidentiality, informed consent, and clinical practices				❑ Staff verbalization ❑ Observation
20. Sensitive and responsive to patients' and coworkers' culture, age, gender, and disabilities				❑ Other
21. Issues regarding the practitioner's physical/mental ability to safely render care				

22. Patient Satisfaction ❑ No comments on file ❑ Complaints ❑ Comments on file: Positive #____ Negative #____ ❑ Trends

Comments (include factor number, as appropriate): _____

_____

_____

_____

_____

_____

_____

_____

_____

Evaluation completed by: _____ Date: _____

Profile reviewed and accepted by: _____ Date: _____

Source: CareLink of Jackson, Jackson, MI

Figure 1.4	Medical staff proctoring policy/procedure

Statement: Upon appointment to the medical/allied health staff (medical staff) each practitioner shall have his or her performance monitored, evaluated, documented, and reported to the medical executive committee (MEC) on an ongoing basis. Focused monitoring and evaluation may be accomplished through proctoring.

Purpose: To define the medical staff procedure and quality improvement process of evaluating and documenting, through direct observation, the performance of practitioners granted clinical privileges at this organization.

Definition of proctoring: The personal presence of an assigned practitioner (proctor) who is designated to provide clinical teaching or to monitor the clinical performance of another practitioner to facilitate quality of care, privileging, performance improvement, or as required by corrective action.

Policy: Focused professional practice evaluations (proctoring) of noncore privileges shall be performed and documented for each practitioner without documented current performance at this organization. The medical director or his or her designee shall, at any time, immediately act upon any reported concern regarding a privileged practitioner's clinical practice or competence. Concerns regarding a practitioner's clinical practice or competence are to be immediately reported to the medical director or clinical service chief.

Candidates for proctoring: Initial applicants, current members requesting new privileges, or medical staff members in need of additional training required for performance improvement or corrective action issues:

1. The practitioner to be proctored is responsible for notifying his or her assigned proctor of each patient whose care is to be evaluated, arranging the time with the proctor for any specific procedure to be proctored, and providing the information requested by the proctor regarding the patient and planned course of treatment.

2. The proctored practitioner will inform the patient that another practitioner may observe and assist in the procedure/course of treatment. Both the proctor and the proctored practitioner's name are to be included on the informed consent form.

3. Monitoring/proctoring of specific procedures shall be performed as required by the clinical service, or as requested by the medical director or clinical service chief. The medical director or clinical service chief will determine the appropriate number of procedures or observations to be proctored.

| Figure 1.4 | Medical staff proctoring policy/procedure (cont.) |

Assignment of a proctor: The medical director or clinical service chief of each involved service may assign, or upon request approve, any appropriately privileged and experienced medical staff member to be a proctor. If a proctor cannot be chosen from the medical staff due to an obvious or perceived potential conflict of interest, the medical director and VP/COO shall agree upon a proctor who may or may not be a current member of another hospital's medical staff. Proctors will not receive compensation directly or indirectly from any patient for this service.

1. The proctor's primary responsibility is to evaluate the proctored practitioner's performance, which may require one or any combination of the following:

    a. The proctor's presence during a specified portion of the procedure (a proctor is permitted to intervene and take any action they find reasonably necessary to avert harm to a patient)

    b. Availability for immediate consultation or concurrent chart review within 24 hours of admission or of the procedure in question

2. Due to the nature of the hospital, proctoring may occur at another hospital, with the approval of the medical director and vice president/chief operating officer (VP/COO), if the same circumstances (equipment/supplies/support) are available at this organization for future performance of the specified procedure. Completion and submission of this organization's approved proctoring form is required.

3. The medical staff office (MSO) shall provide each proctor with the approved proctoring evaluation form and a confidential return envelope, as needed. Extra copies are available in the MSO/library. Evaluations shall be submitted to the MSO within 48 hours of the proctoring. Proctoring evaluations are peer review documents and will remain confidential in accordance with other medical staff peer review information.

Proctoring duration:

1. The medical director, clinical service chief, or the MEC shall determine the length of time allowed for the proctoring process to be completed, which may vary due to the nature of the hospital, the proctored practitioner's specialty (e.g., podiatry), or the reason proctoring is required.

2. A medical staff member may request an extension of time to complete the proctoring if he or she has not had a sufficient number of cases to satisfy the proctoring requirements.

3. With the exception of proctoring required by corrective action, the medical director or clinical service chief, upon consultation with the medical director, may, at any time, determine that sufficient proctoring has occurred to demonstrate competence in the clinical privilege(s) under review and may terminate a proctoring requirement before the designated number of cases have been observed. In such a case, the medical director or clinical service chief shall notify the proctored physician and the MEC in writing of this determination.

4. The MSO shall provide the medical director and clinical service chief(s) with a cumulative list of each practitioner's proctoring as it progresses.

Figure 1.4	Medical staff proctoring policy/procedure (cont.)

Quality of care issues: It is the organization's policy that quality concerns regarding patient care be addressed as they arise to provide continuous quality patient care and safety and to ensure favorable clinical outcomes. A quality concern regarding any practitioner may be raised by medical or allied health staff or nursing staff or through the performance improvement process. If a collegial approach to the concern is not effective (see Concurrent quality concerns policy), the concerned party will file a written report with the MSO.

Quality of care issues should be reported using an occurrence reporting form, disruptive behavior reporting form, or patient grievance flow sheet. These forms are available on each nursing unit and through the MSO. All reports are processed in accordance with medical staff bylaws and the concurrent quality concerns, medical review process, and peer review policies. Any evaluation referencing peer review or quality concern issues shall be submitted to the MEC during its next meeting; however, the medical director or his or her designee shall, at any time, immediately act upon any reported concern regarding a practitioner's clinical practice or competence.

Temporary privileges: Special requirements of supervision and reporting may be imposed upon any individual granted temporary clinical privileges. Notice of any failure by the individual to comply with such special requirements may result in immediate termination of privileges.

Issue resolution: The organization supports the medical staff in addressing all quality of care concerns regarding practitioners through a nonbiased and nonpunitive process by which all provider-related occurrences are reviewed and documented and appropriate action is taken. The medical director and MEC shall perform such oversight, with input from the clinical services. The peer review policy establishes the process and circumstances by which medical staff quality of care reviews, such as peer review and unresolved complaints, may be resolved in a nonpunitive atmosphere that promotes education, performance improvement, and favorable clinical outcomes. Circumstances requiring peer review are delineated in the peer review policy.

Failure of any medical staff member to satisfactorily complete required proctoring will be reviewed and acted upon in accordance with the procedures set forth in bylaws articles VI.D–F.

Approved: _____   _____

            Medical director   Date

_____   _____

            Vice president/Chief operating officer   Date

Source: CareLink of Jackson, Jackson, MI

Figure 1.5	Proctoring evaluation form

Note: *This document serves as attachment B to the Focused professional practice evaluation: Policy/Procedure (Figure 1.1). An individual proctor completes this form on a selected case.*

Procedure date: _____ Medical records number: _____ Practitioner: _____

Proctor: _____ Phone number: _____

Diagnosis: _____

Procedure: _____

Please complete the following based upon your direct observation, discussion with the practitioner being proctored, and review of the patient's record. Please submit this completed form to the medical staff office within 48 hours of proctoring this procedure.

Procedure (*comment required on last page)	Yes	No*	N/A
1. Was there preprocedure justification for the proposed procedure?			
2. Was there appropriate preprocedure discussion with the patient/family?			
3. Was this procedure the most appropriate for this patient?			
4. Was the practitioner's proposed technique appropriate?			
5. Was the practitioner's performance within the accepted standard of care?			
6. Was the practitioner's knowledge of the equipment acceptable?			
7. Was the practitioner knowledgeable of possible complications?			
8. Were complications recognized promptly and dealt with appropriately?			
9. Were the practitioner's postoperative care and orders appropriate?			
10. Was the practitioner's choice of drugs for this procedure appropriate?			
11. Was the practitioner's use of blood and blood components appropriate?			
12. Was all necessary information (history, progress/operative notes, summary) recorded by the practitioner in a timely manner in the medical record?			
13. Was this information recorded legibly?			
14. Were the practitioner's entries in the record informative and appropriate?			
15. Was this procedure completed successfully?			

General (*comment required on last page)	Superior	Average	Poor*
1. Basic medical knowledge			
2. Clinical judgment			
3. Professional attitude (ethical, compassionate, accountable)			
4. Communication skills (clear, concise, verbal/nonverbal)			
5. Interaction with patient/family (respectful, compassionate)			
6. Interaction with staff (respectful, responsive)			
7. Recordkeeping (appropriate, legible, timely)			

Figure 1.5	Proctoring evaluation form (cont.)

Did you intervene at any time to prevent possible harm to the patient? ❑ Yes* ❑ No
Complications/response (as applicable): _____
_____
_____
_____

I rate this practitioner's skill and competence in performing this procedure as:
❑ Superior   ❑ Within the standard of care   ❑ Needs improvement*
❑ Unacceptable because: _____
_____
_____
_____

❑ Unable to evaluate because: _____
_____
_____
_____

*Comments (reference question number, as applicable): _____
_____
_____
_____
_____

Signature of proctor: _____ Date: _____

> Some organizations include a citation at the bottom of these forms that note the state statute that protects the information on the form to reduce or prevent discovery of the contents of the document.

This is a confidential professional peer review and quality assurance document of this organization. It is protected from disclosure pursuant to the provisions of MCL 333.21513, MCL 333.21515, MCL 333.20175(8), MCL 330.1143a, MCL 331.531, and MCL 331.533. Unauthorized disclosure or duplication is absolutely prohibited.

Source: CareLink of Jackson, Jackson, MI

Figure 1.6	Proctoring summary report

Note: *This organization utilizes the same review criteria, and thus the same form, for the initial applicant, requested new privileges, performance improvement, and corrective action. This form is a summary of the findings from the individual proctoring evaluation form (Figure 1.3).*

Practitioner: _____

Clinical service/specialty: _____

Proctor(s): _____

Procedure: _____

Cases proctored: _____ Cases required: _____

Proctoring for: ☒ Initial Applicant (noncore privilege)   ☐ New privilege request
☐ Performance improvement   ☐ Corrective action

Evelution summary	Yes	No*	N/A
Were all procedures completed successfully?			
Was the accepted standard of care achieved/surpassed for each procedure?			
Were all procedures completed without complication?			
Were complications dealt with promptly and appropriately?			
Did a proctor have to intervene at any time to prevent harm to the patient?			
Were any areas for improvement identified?			
Was all documentation completed appropriately and in a timely manner?			
Was any unacceptable behavior reported by any proctor?			

* Information from proctoring evaluation forms or other information submitted by the proctor(s):

I verify that this report was completed using information submitted by the proctor(s) listed above:

_____   _____
Medical director   Date

Figure 1.6	Proctoring summary report (cont.)

Recommendation:

I verify that I have reviewed the proctoring evaluation forms, this report, and all available pertinent information regarding this practitioner. Based upon this review I recommend:

❑ Approval of this practitioner for unrestricted performance of the procedure noted here.

❑ Continued proctoring for this procedure due to: _____

_____

❑ Voluntary withdrawal of this privilege until approved additional training has been completed and supporting documentation submitted for review. Upon acceptance of said documentation, the practitioner may reapply for this privilege and must agree to participate in any required proctoring.

❑ Other: _____

_____

_____   _____
Medical director   Date

_____   _____
Clinical service chief   Date

Source: CareLink of Jackson, Jackson, MI

Figure 1.7	Proctor letter

Date: _____

Name of proctor: _____

Address: _____

RE: Proctoring for [*practitioner's name*]

Dear [*proctor*],

We appreciate your expertise and willingness to serve as [*proctored practitioner's name*] proctor for [*procedure name*]. Our medical director has advised the proctoree of your willingness to serve and reminded the proctored practitioner that it is [*his/her*] responsibility to contact you and arrange a suitable time for you to proctor [*him/her*] for each procedure.

Enclosed you will find a copy of our proctoring policy, along with a supply of proctoring evaluation forms and confidential return envelopes. Please review the policy and familiarize yourself with the evaluation form prior to your first scheduled procedure with the proctored practitioner.

Based on your direct observation, discussion with the practitioner being proctored, and review of the patient's record, you will need to complete an evaluation form for each case you proctor and submit it to the medical staff office within 48 hours of the procedure.

Again, thank you for agreeing to serve as one of [*proctored practitioner's name*] proctors. Please contact the medical director or myself if you have any questions or concerns.

Sincerely,

Medical staff coordinator

Source: CareLink of Jackson, Jackson, MI

Figure 1.8	Letter for the proctored practitioner

Date: _____

Name of proctor: _____

Address: _____

RE: Proctoring for [*practitioner's name*]

Dear [*proctored practitioner*],

We are pleased to notify you that [*name of proctor*] has agreed to [*his/her*] appointment as one of your proctors for [*name of procedure*]. [*Name of proctor*] is aware of [*his/her*] responsibilities as a proctor and that it is your responsibility to contact [*him/her*] in advance to arrange a suitable time for each procedure.

Enclosed you will find copies of our proctoring policy and proctoring evaluation form. Please review the policy and familiarize yourself with the evaluation form prior to your first proctored procedure. Proctors will evaluate care based on direct observation, discussions with you, and review of your patient(s) record(s). Proctors are responsible for completing an evaluation form for each case they proctor and submitting it to the medical staff office within 48 hours of the procedure. Each proctor has been sent a copy of the policy, along with a supply of evaluation forms and confidential return envelopes.

Thank you for your continued cooperation with this quality improvement process. Please feel free to contact the medical director or myself if you have any questions or concerns.

Sincerely,

Medical staff coordinator

Source: CareLink of Jackson, Jackson, MI

Chapter 2

Mercy Medical Center, Nampa, ID

Mercy Medical Center is a rural acute care hospital accredited by The Joint Commission (formerly JCAHO). It has 152 beds and is served by a 274-member medical staff. The medical center has received a number of quality awards, including ones from BlueCross of Idaho and *USA Today*. Mercy's medical services are provided at Mercy Medical Center and the hospital's other facilities: Mercy North Health Center, Mercy Home Health and Hospice, and the Mercy Family Birthing Center.

Sue Salyer, CPMSM, medical staff coordinator at Mercy Medical Center, says that her organization adapted existing documents to meet The Joint Commission's new focused professional practice evaluation (FPPE) standards. The greatest difficulty Salyer says she has faced over the years is medical staff participation in proctoring and collecting completed documents from practitioners. Some of the reasons for these difficulties include a waning interest in medical staff culture on the part of some practitioners and a general sense of being overburdened with paperwork. Additionally, Mercy has seen a drop in the number of physicians practicing at the hospital and has recently started a hospitalist program, two other factors that will affect the fulfilment of medical staff responsiblities.

In response to these challenges, Mercy developed a corrective action plan to improve proctoring participation. Now practitioners are subject to an automatic suspension of privileges if their proctoring is not completed or the proctoring forms are not returned. If a practitioner is having difficulty getting the proctor to complete the proctoring, he or she may ask the department chair for a new proctor. However, Salyer says that the biggest proctoring burden still resides with the medical staff office, which must monitor the process, including organizing the charts for review and reminding the practitioner and his or her proctor of their FPPE responsibilities.

Figure 2.1	Focused professional practice evaluation policy and procedure

Purpose: To define the process for focused professional practice evaluation (FPPE) of medical staff members at Mercy Medical Center.

Policy: FPPE is conducted to assist the medical staff in assessing current clinical competence of medical staff members at Mercy Medical Center under the following circumstances:

1. Initially requested privileges of all new medical staff members

2. Current medical staff members seeking additional privileges or privileges to perform new or rarely performed procedures prior to granting of the privilege to independently perform requested procedures

3. When questions arise regarding a practitioner's professional performance that may affect the provision of safe, high-quality patient care

FPPE for initially requested privileges and for new or additional privileges:

Evaluation period: The evaluation period for initially requested procedures/admissions of new appointees shall be determined by the appropriate department. If a proctor is assigned, the proctor will continue to act in an advisory capacity to the appointee throughout his or her provisional year. The evaluation period may be extended for a period not to exceed one additional year.

The evaluation period for new or additional privileges shall be determined by the appropriate department or credentials committee on a case-by-case basis.

Terms of evaluation: Approved evaluation methods may include chart review (both concurrent and retrospective), monitoring clinical practice patterns, direct observation, external peer review, discussion with other individuals involved in the care of each patient (e.g., consulting physicians, assistants at surgery, nursing or administrative personnel) and may include an evaluation of the physician's ability to work harmoniously with others and of the physician's interpersonal skills with peers, nursing staff, ancillary personnel, and hospital administration.

The terms of evaluation may vary from one department to another (as predetermined by each department); however, procedures crossing specialty lines should have uniform evaluation requirements. The minimum number of cases/procedures to be reviewed shall not be altered except in cases of extenuating circumstances.

Duties and responsibilities of department chairs: Each medical staff department chair shall be responsible for:

1. Assisting the department in establishing a minimum number of cases/procedures to be evaluated and determining when a proctor must be present. When there are privileges that cross specialty lines, the credentials committee shall determine the minimum number of cases/procedures to be reviewed.

| Figure 2.1 | Focused professional practice evaluation policy and procedure (cont.) |

2. Identifying the names of medical staff members eligible to serve as proctors and assigning of proctors as noted below.

3. If at any time during a proctoring period, the proctor notifies the department chair that he or she has concerns about the practitioner's competency to perform specific clinical privileges or care related to a specific patient(s), based on the recommendations of the proctor, the department chair shall then review the medical records of the patient(s) treated by the practitioner being proctored and shall take one of the following actions:

    a. Intervene and adjudicate the conflict if the proctor and the practitioner disagree as to what constitutes appropriate care for a patient
    b. Refer the case(s) for peer review pursuant to the peer review policy
    c. Make one of the following recommendations to the medical executive committee (MEC):
        1) Additional or revised proctoring requirements should be imposed upon the practitioner
        2) Corrective action should be undertaken pursuant to the corrective action plan

Duties and responsibilities of the medical staff office (MSO): The MSO shall:

1. Send a letter to the practitioner being evaluated and to any assigned proctor containing the following information:

    a. Evaluation requirements as predetermined by the department or credentials committee
    b. The name and telephone numbers of the practitioner being proctored and the proctor, as well as proctoring forms to be completed
    c. A copy of the FPPE policy and procedure

2. Develop a mechanism (in coordination with health information department or performance improvement department) to track admissions, procedures, and clinical practice patterns of the practitioner being evaluated

3. For practitioners being proctored,

    a. Provide information to appropriate hospital departments about practitioners being proctored, including the name of the proctor and a supply of proctoring forms as needed
    b. Periodically contact both the proctor and practitioner being proctored to ensure that proctoring and chart reviews are being conducted as required

4. Periodically submit a report to the appropriate departments or MEC of evaluation activity for all practitioners being evaluated

5. At the conclusion of the evaluation period, submit a summary report on each practitioner being evaluated to the credentials committee and MEC

Figure 2.1	Focused professional practice evaluation policy and procedure (cont.)

Proctoring procedure:

Assignment of proctor: The department chair will appoint a proctor from a list of medical staff members of that specific department. To the extent possible, a proctor should be qualified and possess credentials similar to the practitioner being proctored.

When the situation exists in which no other physician is qualified or credentialed to serve as a proctor or a conflict of interest has been declared, an outside proctor may be retained. An outside proctor may be granted temporary privileges to serve in a proctoring capacity.

Duties and responsibilities of practitioners being proctored: Practitioners being proctored shall:

1. Notify the proctor of each case where care is to be evaluated and, when required, do so in sufficient time to allow the proctor to observe or review concurrently. For elective surgical or invasive procedures for which direct observation is required, the practitioner must secure agreement from the proctor to attend the procedure. In an emergency, the practitioner may arrange for proctoring by another member of the medical staff with appropriate independent privileges or admit and treat the patient; however, the practitioner must notify the proctor as soon as reasonably possible.

2. Have the prerogative of requesting from the department chair a change of proctor if disagreements with or incomplete proctoring duties by the current proctor may adversely affect his or her ability to satisfactorily complete the proctorship. The department chair will make a recommendation on this matter to the MEC for final action.

3. Inform the proctor of any unusual incident(s) associated with his or her patients.

4. Ensure documentation of the satisfactory completion of his or her proctorship, including the completion and delivery of proctorship forms and the summary proctor report to the MSO. The proctoring period will automatically extend for up to three months if the proctorship forms and the summary proctor report are not completed and submitted at the end of the initial proctoring period. If the proctorship forms and summary proctor report are not completed and submitted to the MSO by the end of a proctoring period extended under this subparagraph 4, the privileges of a provisional appointee subject to proctoring, or the additional or new privileges which are the subject of proctoring for any other member of the medical staff, shall be automatically suspended. Failure to obtain submission of completed proctorship forms and a summary proctor report prior to the time for submission of the physician's next reappointment application shall be treated as a voluntary relinquishment of the privileges that were subject to proctoring.

Figure 2.1	Focused professional practice evaluation policy and procedure (cont.)

Duties and responsibilities of the proctor: The proctor shall:

1. As predetermined by the department or credentials committee:

    a. Directly observe the procedure being performed
    b. Concurrently observe medical management for the medical admission
    c. Retrospectively review the completed medical record following discharge

2. Complete proctoring forms and ensure their confidentiality and delivery to the MSO

3. Submit a summary proctor report at the conclusion of the proctoring period

4. If at any time during the proctoring period the proctor has concerns about the practitioner's competency to perform specific clinical privileges or care related to a specific patient(s), the proctor shall promptly notify the department chair and may recommend that:

    a. The department chair intervene and adjudicate the conflict if the proctor and the practitioner disagree as to what constitutes appropriate care for a patient
    b. The department chair review the case for possible peer review, pursuant to the peer review policy
    c. Additional or revised proctoring requirements be imposed upon the practitioner until the proctor can make an informed judgment and recommendation regarding the clinical performance of the individual being proctored
    d. The appointee's continued appointment and clinical privileges be referred to the MEC

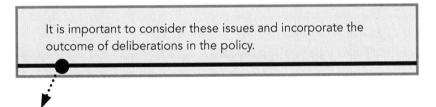

It is important to consider these issues and incorporate the outcome of deliberations in the policy.

Liability of proctor: A practitioner serving solely as a proctor, for the purpose of assessing and reporting on the competence of another practitioner, is an agent of the hospital. The proctor shall receive no compensation directly or indirectly from any patient for this service, and he or she shall have no duty to the patient to intervene if the care provided by the proctored practitioner is deficient or appears to be deficient. The proctor, or any other practitioner, however, may nonetheless render emergency medical care to the patient for medical complications arising from the care provided by the proctored practitioner. The hospital will defend and indemnify any practitioner who is subjected to a claim or suit arising out of his or her acts or omissions in the role of proctor.

Completion of proctorship: At the end of the proctoring period, the proctor shall provide a summary report to the department chair and credentials committee that shall include one or more of the following:

Figure 2.1	Focused professional practice evaluation policy and procedure (cont.)

a. Whether a sufficient number of cases done at Mercy Medical Center have been presented for review to properly evaluate the clinical privileges requested

b. If a sufficient number of cases have not been presented for review, whether, in the proctor's opinion, the proctoring period or provisional appointment should be extended

c. If a sufficient number of cases have been presented to properly evaluate the clinical privileges requested, a report concerning the qualifications and competence of the practitioner being proctored to independently exercise these privileges

d. For provisional appointees, make a recommendation for permanent membership and continued clinical privileges as requested, recommend an additional proctoring period or continued provisional staff status not to exceed an additional year, or not recommend permanent membership and continued clinical privileges as requested

e. For new or additional privileges, make a recommendation to independently perform the requested privileges, recommend an additional proctoring period, or not recommend continued clinical privileges as requested

FPPE for physician performance issues:

FPPE shall be conducted when questions arise regarding a practitioner's professional performance that may affect the provision of safe, high-quality patient care that have been identified through the peer review process, ongoing feedback reports, or pursuant to the corrective action plan.

Triggers that may initiate this process include but are not limited to:

a. Significant deviation from accepted standards of practice

b. Adverse or negative performance trends

c. Repeated failure to follow hospital policy

d. Significant staff or patient complaint(s)

e. Upon recommendation of the department chair pursuant to section IV.B. of the peer review policy

The determination to assign a period of focused monitoring should be based on the practitioner's current clinical competence, practice behavior, and ability to perform the privileges at issue. Other existing privileges in good standing should not be affected by this decision.

The terms, methods, and duration of the evaluation period shall be determined by MEC.

Source: Mercy Medical Center, Nampa, ID.

Figure 2.2	Emergency department proctor report

Retrospective chart review protected under Idaho code section 39:1392

Date of ED visit: _____ Medical record number/patient name: _____

Date of this review: _____ Diagnosis/presenting complaint: _____

_____

_____

Proctored practitioner's name: _____

Proctor name: _____

Evaluate in terms of completeness and accuracy	Acceptable	Marginal (explain)	Unacceptable (explain)	N/A
Diagnostic work-up				
Patient was triaged and seen in a timely manner	❏	❏	❏	❏
Emergency notes are complete and appropriate to patient's condition	❏	❏	❏	❏
Diagnostic tests are appropriate (lab and x-ray)	❏	❏	❏	❏
Diagnostic procedures are appropriate	❏	❏	❏	❏
Comments: _____				
Patient management				
Consultation used appropriately	❏	❏	❏	❏
Ancillary services used appropriately	❏	❏	❏	❏
Abnormal lab and x-ray results are recognized/followed-up	❏	❏	❏	❏
Complications are managed appropriately	❏	❏	❏	❏
Drug and therapeutic regimens meet accepted standards	❏	❏	❏	❏
Monitoring of patient's condition is appropriate	❏	❏	❏	❏
ED length of stay is within acceptable standards	❏	❏	❏	❏
Comments: _____				

Figure 2.2	Emergency department proctor report (cont.)

Disposition				
Justification for admission documented	❏	❏	❏	❏
Placement (transfer, home, other) appropriate and reflected in chart	❏	❏	❏	❏
Patient education/instruction (diet, medications, follow-up, level of activity, etc.) is appropriate and reflected in chart	❏	❏	❏	❏

Comments: _____

_____

_____

Overall performance				
Interaction with colleagues, staff, and patient	❏	❏	❏	❏
Overall impression of care provided	❏	❏	❏	❏

Comments: _____

_____

_____

Is there any aspect of this patient's treatment and follow-up with which you are uneasy or uncomfortable?   ❏ No   ❏ Yes   If yes, please explain: _____

_____

_____

_____

Proctor's signature: _____ Date: _____

Please return to medical staff office immediately following review.

Source: Mercy Medical Center, Nampa, ID.

Figure 2.3	Surgical proctor report

Please circle one: Direct/concurrent review   Retrospective chart review

Protected under Idaho code section 39:1392

Date of this review: _____   Medical record number: _____
Poctored practitioner: _____   Proctor: _____
Diagnosis: _____
Procedure: _____

Evaluate in terms of completeness and accuracy	Acceptable	Marginal (explain)	Unacceptable (explain)	N/A
Preoperative work-up				
H&Ps are complete, accurate, and in chart	❑	❑	❑	❑
Consent(s) are appropriate and signed	❑	❑	❑	❑
Lab and x-ray are appropriate	❑	❑	❑	❑
Progress notes regarding planned procedure are complete	❑	❑	❑	❑
Preoperative indication for surgery	❑	❑	❑	❑

Comments: _____
_____
_____

Intraoperative phase				
Punctuality of surgeon/anesthetist	❑	❑	❑	❑
Technical skill	❑	❑	❑	❑
Knowledge of procedure	❑	❑	❑	❑
Blood loss	❑	❑	❑	❑

Comments: _____
_____
_____

Surgical judgment				
Completeness and degree/extent of resection; degree to which operation conforms to acceptable practices	❑	❑	❑	❑
Conduct in operating room	❑	❑	❑	❑

Comments: _____
_____

Figure 2.3	Surgical proctor report (cont.)

Postoperative phase

Preop diagnosis and postop findings coincide	❑	❑	❑	❑
Postoperative care	❑	❑	❑	❑
Operative report complete, accurate and timely	❑	❑	❑	❑
Complications (if any) are recognized and managed appropriately	❑	❑	❑	❑
Discharge plans (including patient instructions) are reflected in chart	❑	❑	❑	❑
Length of stay is within acceptable standards	❑	❑	❑	❑
Surgery is justified by pathology reports	❑	❑	❑	❑

Comments: _____
_____
_____

Overall performance

Interaction with colleagues, staff, and patient	❑	❑	❑	❑
Overall impression of care provided	❑	❑	❑	❑

Comments: _____
_____
_____

Is there any aspect of this patient's treatment and follow-up with which you are uneasy or uncomfortable?   ❑ No   ❑ Yes   If yes, please explain: _____
_____
_____
_____

Proctor's signature: _____ Date: _____

Please return to medical staff office immediately following review.

Source: Mercy Medical Center, Nampa, ID.

| Figure 2.4 | Performance feedback process for mid-level practitioners |

Note: *It is important for organizations to realize that FPPE pertains to all privileged practitioners, not only to medical staff members.*

Purpose/scope: The purpose of this process is to monitor performance/competency of midlevel practitioners to measure and continually improve performance and provide ongoing assessment in a measurable way. The findings will be reported to the board of directors after the first provisional year and at least every other year thereafter.

Background: Physician assistants (PA) and nurse practitioners (NP) are midlevel practitioners at Mercy Medical Center and do not function independently in accordance with the hospital's policy. Physician supervision is outlined in the delegation of services agreement/supervising physician agreement on file in the medical staff office.

Guidelines:

A. Provisional Year

Performance feedback during the provisional year will occur as follows:

1) Five cases will be reviewed each quarter and the results reported to the department chair.
2) The supervising physician and department director(s) will be asked to provide an evaluation quarterly. The department chair will be notified of any adverse findings.
3) At the end of the provisional year, quarterly reports will be compiled and aggregate information will be reported to the department chair, credentials committee, medical executive committee, and the board of directors.

B. Ongoing Evaluation

After the provisional year, ongoing evaluation will occur as follows:

1) Cases are screened for peer review indicators. If a midlevel practitioner was involved in a case that is identified for peer review, the midlevel practitioner will be asked to attend the meeting and participate in the peer review.
2) If a finding is attributed to the midlevel practitioner, the case will be tracked through the peer review system and reported at the time of reappointment.
3) At the end of each two-year reappointment period, the supervising physician and department director(s) will be asked to provide an evaluation.
4) The medical staff office will aggregate the information and report to the department chair who will make a recommendation for reappointment to the credentials committee, medical executive committee, and the board of directors.

Measures: Performance evaluation during the provisional year will cover the following dimensions of performance: technical quality, service quality, patient safety, resource utilization, peer and coworker relationships, and citizenship.

The following indicators will be used to measure provider performance against the dimensions of performance. (Indicators in bold will be collected by PI. Other indicators will be evidenced through an evaluation tool completed by department directors/supervising physician):

Figure 2.4	Performance feedback pocess for mid-level practitioners (cont).

A. Technical Quality
   1) **Case volumes by diagnosis/Diagnosis-related group**
   2) **Readmission rates**
   3) **Complication rates**
   4) **Number of cases sent to peer review**
   5) **Mortality rates**
   6) **Number/types of incident reports**
   7) Skills for scope of practice requested/practices within scope
   8) Physician oversight

B. Service Quality
   1) How well providers deliver care to their patients
   2) Use of scripting/participation in other customer service initiatives
   3) Approach/rapport with patients and families
   4) Appropriate communication with the healthcare team
   5) Responding to pages/requests in a timely manner
   6) Timeliness and accuracy of dictation/medical record completion

C. Patient Safety
   1) **Legible, complete, timely, and accurate medical records**
   2) **Use of prohibited abbreviations**
   3) Compliance with universal precautions/hand hygiene

D. Resource Utilization
   1) Under-/over-utilization of medications/equipment
   2) **Number of denials**
   3) **Number of avoidable days**

E. Peer and Coworker Relationships
   1) Mutual respect among the heathcare team
   2) Interpersonal relationships/cooperation with other disciplines
   3) **Number of complaints**
   4) Identifies themselves as PA/NP
   5) Wears a name badge in the facility

F. Citizenship
   1) **Attends meetings when a peer review case is discussed**
   2) Maintains patient confidentiality
   3) Supports the mission/vision of the hospital

Source: Mercy Medical Center, Nampa, ID.

| Figure 2.5 | Performance feedback algorithm for mid-level practitioners |

Note: *It is important to note regarding the box stating "PI conducts chart review and completes evaluation" that if a concern is raised during the review, the department chair is immediately notified.*

Regarding the box "Department Directors complete evaluation," it is important to note that, at this hospital, department directors are hospital service line directors.

Each quarter medical staff office sends PI and department directors a list of names of mid-level practitioners during their provisional year

PI conducts chart review and completes evaluation

Department directors complete evaluation

Send the completed evaluation back to the medical staff office

The medical staff office will send PI and department director evaluations to supervising physician

Supervising physician completes evaluation and sends it back to the medical staff office

Adverse findings

No Adverse findings

Department chair reviews adverse findings

Medical staff office reviews all evaluations for adverse findings

Evaluations reviewed annually by department chair and credentials committee

Source: Mercy Medical Center, Nampa, ID.

Figure 2.6	Nurse midwife proctor report

Protected under Idaho code section 39:1392

Date of this review: _____ Medical record number: _____

Midwife proctored: _____ Proctor: _____

Was this a low-risk delivery? ☐ Yes ☐ No If no, please explain: _____

_____

_____

Evaluate in terms of completeness and accuracy	Acceptable	Marginal (explain)	Unacceptable (explain)	N/A
Predelivery work-up				
Sponsoring physician notified and physician's name documented in chart at time of admission	☐	☐	☐	☐
H&Ps are complete, accurate and on chart	☐	☐	☐	☐
Consent(s) are appropriate and signed	☐	☐	☐	☐
Ancillary services are used appropriately	☐	☐	☐	☐
Progress notes are complete and timely	☐	☐	☐	☐
Comments: _____ _____ _____				
OB management				
Predelivery management	☐	☐	☐	☐
Labor management	☐	☐	☐	☐
Anesthesia management	☐	☐	☐	☐
Newborn management	☐	☐	☐	☐
Postdelivery management	☐	☐	☐	☐
Conduct in labor and delivery room	☐	☐	☐	☐
Comments: _____ _____ _____				

| Figure 2.6 | Nurse midwife proctor report (cont.) |

Surgical judgment

Completeness and degree/extent of resection; degree to which operation conforms to acceptable practices	❑	❑	❑	❑
Conduct in operating room	❑	❑	❑	❑

Comments: _____
_____
_____

Patient management

Clinical judgment: Degree to which delivery conforms to acceptable practices	❑	❑	❑	❑
Technical skill: Complications (if any) are recognized and managed appropriately	❑	❑	❑	❑
Discharge plans (including patient instructions) are reflected in chart	❑	❑	❑	❑
Appropriate collaboration/consultation with or referral to sponsoring physician/group	❑	❑	❑	❑

Comments: _____
_____
_____

Overall performance

Interaction with colleagues, staff, and patient	❑	❑	❑	❑
Overall impression of care provided	❑	❑	❑	❑

Comments: _____
_____
_____

Is there any aspect of this patient's treatment and follow-up with which you are uneasy or uncomfortable?   ❑ No   ❑ Yes   If yes, please explain: _____
_____
_____
_____

Proctor's signature: _____ Date: _____

Please return to medical staff office immediately following review.

Source: Mercy Medical Center, Nampa, ID.

Figure 2.7	Proctoring by department

In addition to the requirements listed here, all proctors will complete a summary review of the proctored physician at the end of one year. Provisional period may be extended no more than one year.

Medical staff departments	Types/numbers of procedures	Method/duration
Anesthesia	1. Three charts per quarter 2. One to two cases per quarter	Concurrent chart review, one year Direct observation of induction and emergence by any anesthesiologist, one year
Emergency	Physicians: Five charts per month for first three months	Physicians: Five charts per month for first three months
Family Practice	1. Three OB deliveries 2. Six C-sections 3. Six tubal ligations 4. Three pediatric admissions 5. Five each for endoscopic procedures 6. 15 medical/surgical/ICU admissions	OB deliveries: Direct observation by proctor/in-house physician with OB privileges, first six months C-section and tubals: Direct observation by OB or family practitioner with appropriate privileges Pediatrics: Concurrent observation/chart review, first six months Endoscopy: Direct observation, first six months (Check endoscopy for whether FP doctor does them; if not, get medicine proctor. Medical/surgical/ICU: concurrent chart review, in first year)

Medicine	1. Five each for endoscopic procedures
	2. Five for each medical subspecialty
	
	Cardiology: proctor determines the number of observed procedures based on training and experience
		Direct observation:
		
		  a. Bronchoscopy (by physician with bronchoscopy privileges), first six months
		  b. Endoscopy: first six months
		
		Each medical subspecialty: Concurrent chart review, if possible. If not possible, review should be completed within 60 days. If the proctor detects a problem, then concurrent review should begin immediately.
		
		Plus: Cardiology: Direct observation

Midlevel practitioners (see midlevel practitioner feedback process)	**Supervised:** PAs/NPs: Five charts per quarter _____ **Sponsored:** Certified nurse midwife: 1. Five charts per quarter 2. Six vaginal deliveries	ED PAs/NPs: Ongoing quarterly review by two ED physicians on rotational schedule. Results shared with PA/NP. Remaining PAs/NPs: Quarterly review for first year (along with quarterly physician and department director evaluations) _____ Chart review: Quarterly for first year (plus physician and department director evaluations) First six vaginal deliveries: Direct observation by active staff physician with OB/GYN privileges

Figure 2.7	Proctoring by department (cont.)	
Obstetrics	All OB and GYN cases, including but not limited to at least: 1. Five C-sections 2. Five hysterectomies 3. Any three hysteroscopic (level II) 4. Any three advanced pelvic laparoscopy (level II and III)	1 and 2: Direct observation as noted and 100% concurrent surgical chart review for first six months. 3 and 4: See list of procedures on individual criteria.
Pathology	1. 100% of all malignancies 2. Random review of 10% of all cases	Slide review: First two months Slide review: First six months
Pediatrics	10 pediatric charts 20 newborn charts All transfers during the first six months	Concurrent chart review: First year Concurrent chart review: First six months
Radiology	1. 20 diagnostic cases 2. 20 interventional procedures 3. Proctoring physicians to meet with chairman to discuss performance	Direct observation or chart review in first year Direct observation or chart review in first year Each quarter
Surgery	Five different surgical procedures with two of the five defined as major surgical procedures Dentists: Three total procedures	Observation: In first year Dentists: One by direct observation: First six months Two by Chart Review: First six months

Source: Mercy Medical Center, Nampa, ID.

Chapter 3

MeritCare Health System, Fargo, ND

MeritCare Health System, a 100-year-old institution, is the largest hospital in North Dakota. It is accredited by The Joint Commission (formerly JCAHO) and affiliated with the University of North Dakota Medical School for the internal medicine residency program. The first procedure performed at MeritCare, originally named St. Luke's Hospital, was an emergency appendectomy; now the organization has grown to include 32 surgical suites in which more than 19,000 surgical cases are performed each year. MeritCare has 583 beds divided between two locations and is served by a medical staff that includes 407 active members, 96 courtesy members, 204 affiliate members, 21 associate (board eligible) members, and one emeritus member.

Aaste Campbell, medical staff coordinator at MeritCare, says that her organization developed new documents to comply with The Joint Commission's focused professional practice evaluation (FPPE) standards rather than adapting existing documents. First, the chief medical officer wrote the department template policy. It was then distributed to the department chairs so they could adapt their own policies to it. Next, these department policies and additional FPPE forms were sent to the credentials committee and medical staff executive committee for approval.

One roadblock MeritCare faced when developing its FPPE policy was dealing with how to evaluate locum tenens. To solve this problem, the organization contacted The Joint Commission directly for clarification. Campbell says the accreditor told MeritCare that locum tenens are not expected to have the same type of proctoring; however, a retrospective review is appropriate.

Figure 3.1	Focused professional practice evaluations

Note: *This organization chose to create a focused professional practice evaluation (FPPE) policy for newly privileged practitioners, thus separating the process from FPPEs that may result from its ongoing physician practice evaluation processes (OPPE). The organization's expanded definition of proctoring under the "Definitions" section is also of interest.*

Purpose: To establish a systematic proctoring process to ensure that there is sufficient information available to confirm the current competence of practitioners who initially request privileges at MeritCare Hospital, as part of a FPPE.

Definitions:

Proctoring: Proctoring includes one or more of the following as part of a FPPE:

- Presentation of cases with planned treatment outlined for treatment concurrence or review of case documentation for treatment concurrence (prospective proctoring)

- Real-time observation of a procedure (concurrent proctoring)

- Review of a case after care has been completed, which may include interviews with personnel involved in the care of the patient (retrospective proctoring)

- Evidence of successful proctoring at another local hospital, subject to the requirements noted below (reciprocal observation)

All other terms shall have the meanings assigned in the medical staff bylaws.

Procedure:

I. Scope: This policy applies to all practitioners who request initial privileges, including initial applicants for medical or professional staff appointment, current members of the medical or professional staff who request additional clinical privileges, and practitioners requesting temporary privileges.

Practitioners requesting membership but not exercising specific privileges do not need to be proctored.

Proctoring as part of a FPPE for practitioners with existing privileges when questions arise regarding a practitioner's ability to provide safe, high-quality patient care as the result of a single incident or during the course of an OPPE or because of infrequent use of specific privileges are outside the scope of this policy. (Please see the OPPE policy).

| Figure 3.1 | Focused professional practice evaluations (cont.) |

For purposes of this policy, in some organizations the functions of an "executive physician partner" might be comperable to a department chair, and the functions of a "managing physician partner" might be comperable to a section chief.

II. Responsibilities of credentials committee, executive physician partner (EPP), managing physician partner (MPP), departments, and committees:

The credentials committee is charged with the responsibility of monitoring compliance with this policy. It accomplishes this oversight by receiving regular reports related to the progress of all practitioners who are required to be proctored, as well as any issues or problems involved in implementing this policy. The credentials committee, with input from the individual departments, shall determine the minimum standards for proctoring duration and numbers. The credentials committee establishes the minimum duration and type of proctoring and ensures that the privilege forms specify the minimum proctoring and that any individual practitioner's privilege delineation form sets forth the number of procedures, if any, to be subject to concurrent proctoring. The appropriate medical staff committee or department will implement changes to improve performance based on results of FPPEs, including proctoring, and will implement practitioner-specific performance improvement plans, if appropriate, for practitioners who complete the FPPE.

The aggregate EPP, or the MPP for those departments without an EPP, shall be responsible for overseeing the proctoring process for all practitioners assigned to the department, as further described below.

The medical staff committees or departments involved with OPPE will provide the credentials committee with data that are systematically collected through the OPPE processes for those practitioners, as appropriate, to confirm current competence during the FPPE period.

III. Proctoring method:

Proctoring may be performed using prospective, concurrent, or retrospective approaches. Practitioner specialists who most often provide cognitive care, as opposed to procedural care, will be evaluated prospectively/retrospectively. Prospective and concurrent proctoring will be used for evaluating practitioners who request privileges to perform various procedures. The appropriate methods for proctoring for each individual practitioner will be determined by the credentials committee based on recommendations from the departments and approved by the medical executive committee (MEC). Certain practitioners who practice at local hospitals may be eligible for reciprocal observation, in lieu of proctoring at the MeritCare Hospital, as noted below.

Figure 3.1	Focused professional practice evaluations (cont.)

IV. Duration of proctoring period:

The initial time period for FPPE proctoring shall be for a period established by the credentials committee, beginning with the practitioner's first admissions or performance of the newly requested privilege. Based on the class of the practitioner (see below), newly granted privileges shall be considered under FPPE either for a specific period of time or for a specific number of cases based on the recommendation of the credentials committee. The proctoring period may be extended by the credentials committee if initial concerns are raised that require further evaluation or if there is insufficient activity during the initial period, provided, however, the total proctoring period may not exceed 12 months.

V. Extent of practitioner experience:

The medical staff will take into account the practitioner's previous experience in determining the approach and extent of proctoring needed to confirm current competence. The practitioner's experience may fall into one of the following classes:

1. Recent graduate from a training program affiliated with MeritCare Health System, where the requested privileges were part of the training program

2. Recent graduate from a training program at another facility, where the requested privileges were part of the training program

3. A practitioner with regular experience exercising the requested privilege of fewer than two years on another medical staff

4. A practitioner with regular experience exercising the requested privilege of more than five years at another medical staff

As guidelines for the departments and credentials committee, the following sets forth the minimum recommended proctoring for practitioners requesting initial privileges:

- Practitioners in class one may need minimal or no proctoring as defined by their respective departments and the credentials committee, since MeritCare has had the opportunity to observe the current competence of the applicant directly.

- Practitioners in classes two and three will have full proctoring as defined by their respective departments and the credentials committee. Such full proctoring may include retrospective evaluation of cases for all class two or three practitioners. If the practitioner is a specialist who performs procedures, the proctoring may include both prospective and concurrent proctoring.

- Practitioners in class four are candidates for minimal proctoring (as defined for class one) or reciprocal observation, unless concerns exist regarding the recent frequency of the use of requested privileges.

Figure 3.1	Focused professional practice evaluations (cont.)

VI. Reciprocal observation:

When a practitioner has insufficient clinical activity at MeritCare Hospital or does not have the type of clinical activity for the requested privilege that is required to be proctored, MeritCare Hospital may accept evidence of successful proctoring from a local hospital. The following hospitals qualify as acceptable local hospitals: Innovis, Altru, MedCenter One, and St. Alexius. The arrangement is acceptable only under the following circumstances:

1. The practitioner required to be proctored is responsible for identifying the local hospital where information may be obtained and to ensure that representatives of the local hospital provide the requested information.

2. The proctor(s) at the local hospital must have privileges at MeritCare Hospital or be eligible for privileges.

3. The practitioner must consent to authorize the local hospital to release copies of his or her proctoring reports or provide a summary of proctoring activities.

4. A physician representative of the medical staff organization of the local hospital must complete an observation evaluation summary form or other documentation acceptable to MeritCare Hospital and forward to the MeritCare Hospital medical staff office (MSO).

5. The local hospital must provide MeritCare Hospital with a copy of the clinical privileges that have been granted to the practitioner who needs evaluation.

It is within the discretion of the EPP to determine whether the observation at the local hospital meets the requirements of MeritCare Hospital. The EPP's decision will be reviewed by the credentials committee, MEC, and the MeritCare Hospital board of directors (referred to as *board* in this document).

VII. Responsibilities of proctors:

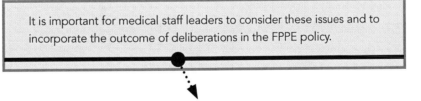

It is important for medical staff leaders to consider these issues and to incorporate the outcome of deliberations in the FPPE policy.

The proctor's role is that of an evaluator—to review and observe cases—not of a supervisor or consultant. The practitioner who is serving solely as a proctor is an agent of the hospital. The proctor receives no compensation directly or indirectly from any patient for this service.

| Figure 3.1 | Focused professional practice evaluations (cont.) |

1. Proctors must be members in good standing of the active medical staff of MeritCare Hospital and have unrestricted privileges to perform any procedure(s) to be concurrently proctored.

2. Proctors shall directly observe the procedure being performed or concurrently proctor medical management for the medial admission and complete appropriate sections of the proctoring form.

3. Proctors will retrospectively review the completed medical record following discharge and complete appropriate sections of the proctoring form.

4. The proctor will monitor the practitioner being proctored from admission to discharge, including the following, as applicable to the patient and the practitioner's specialty:

- History and physical
- Diagnosis and justification of same
- Proposed treatment or procedure and its indications
- Continuity of care provided to the patients
- Appropriateness of tests, procedures, and medications prescribed
- Appropriate use of consultants
- Appropriateness of length of stay
- Adequacy and legibility of progress notes
- Adequacy of operative notes where appropriate
- Discharge summary
- Timely completion of medical records
- Appropriately signed consents
- Technical skills/knowledge (as appropriate)
- Use of blood and blood components
- Punctuality and conduct in OR
- Pre- and postoperative care
- Management of complications

5. The proctor will ensure the confidentiality of the proctoring results and forms. The proctor will deliver the completed forms to the MeritCare Hospital MSO.

6. A summary report will be submitted at the conclusion of the proctoring period.

Figure 3.1	Focused professional practice evaluations (cont.)

7. If at any time during the proctoring period the proctor has concerns about the practitioner's competency to perform specific clinical privileges or care related to a specific patient(s), the proctor shall promptly notify the department EPP or MPP for those departments that do not have an EPP. One of the following may be recommended:

   a. The EPP or MPP will intervene and adjudicate the conflict if the proctor and the practitioner disagree as to what constitutes appropriate care for the patient.

   b. The EPP or MPP will review the case for possible peer review at the next department meeting.

   c. Additional or revised proctoring requirements may be imposed upon the practitioner until the proctor can make an informed judgment and recommendation regarding the clinical performance of the individual being proctored.

   d. A precautionary suspension may be imposed by the EPP or MPP if the failure to take such action may result in imminent danger to the health or safety of any individual or may interfere with the orderly operation of the hospital, in accordance with the medical staff bylaws.

   e. Referral of the practitioner's continued appointment and clinical privileges to the MeritCare Hospital MEC may be made.

> This organization has determined that serving as a proctor is an obligation of all staff members and has identified potential consequences for refusing to serve.

8. It is the responsibility of all members of the active medical staff within each department to serve as proctors when asked to do so. Refusal to accept proctor assignment or to fulfill service as a proctor may result in corrective action.

9. In addition to specialty- and privilege-specific issues, proctoring will also address the six general competencies of practitioner performance: technical/clinical quality, service quality, patient safety, resource use, relations, and citizenship, to the extent observed in the course of the proctoring.

VIII. Responsibilities of executive partners or managing physician partners:

The EPP (or MPP, when there is no EPP for the department) shall be responsible for the following:

1. Assigning proctors as noted earlier or serve as proctors.

2. Helping establish the minimum number of cases or procedures to be proctored and determining the times when the proctor must be present. Where there are inter-departmental privileges, the credentials committee shall determine the minimum number of cases or procedures to be reviewed.

Figure 3.1	Focused professional practice evaluations (cont.)

3. Reviewing the medical records of the patient(s) treated by the practitioner being proctored if, at any time during the proctoring period, the proctor notifies the EPP or MPP that he or she has concerns about the practitioner's competency to perform specific clinical privileges or care related to a specific patient, based on the recommendation of the proctor. The EPP or MPP shall then do one of the actions noted in the previous section regarding responsibilities of proctors, subsections 7 a–e.

IX. Responsibilities of the practitioners being proctored:

1. The practitioner shall notify the proctor of each case in which care is to be evaluated and, when required, do so in sufficient time to enable the proctor to conduct concurrent proctoring. For elective surgical or invasive procedures where concurrent proctoring is required, the practitioner must secure agreement from the proctor to attend and observe the procedure.

2. The practitioner shall provide the proctor with information about the patient's clinical history; pertinent physical findings, lab, and x-ray results; the planned course of treatment or management; and direct delivery of a copy of all histories and physicals, operative reports, consultations, and discharge summaries documented by the proctored practitioner to the proctor.

> An important aspect to consider in advance of placing a new physician on ER call.

3. Practitioners who are initially appointed to the medical staff may not serve alone—that is, without the proctor—in the emergency center call schedule or on call until all required prospective or concurrent observations and retrospective evaluations have been completed and the practitioner has been approved to be on-call by the department's EPP or MPP and the credentials committee chair/designee.

4. The practitioner shall have the prerogative of requesting from the EPP or MPP a change of proctor if disagreements with the current proctor adversely affects his or her ability to complete the proctorship timely and satisfactorily. The EPP or MPP will make recommendations to the credentials committee for final action.

5. The practitioner shall inform the proctor of any unusual incidents associated with his or her patients.

6. The practitioner will ensure documentation of the satisfactory completion of his or her proctorship, including the completion and delivery of proctorship forms and the summary proctor report to the MSO. The proctoring period will be automatically

| Figure 3.1 | Focused professional practice evaluations (cont.) |

extended if the summary proctor report is not completed and submitted at the end of the initial proctoring period. The automatic extension under this section shall be until the date that is three months from the expiration of the initial period or the date that is 12 months from the commencement of the initial period, whichever date is earlier.

7. If the summary proctor report is not completed and submitted to the MSO when due, or the practitioner otherwise fails to complete the proctoring requirements prior to the expiration of the proctoring period, the additional or new privileges that are the subject of proctoring shall be deemed to be voluntarily relinquished by the practitioner and the practitioner shall immediately stop exercising said privileges.

X. Procedural rights: Failure to meet FPPE/proctoring requirements:

1. If a practitioner's appointment or clinical privileges are deemed to be voluntarily relinquished for failure to complete proctoring requirements, the practitioner shall be notified in writing before a report of that voluntary relinquishment is made to the board.

2. As part of the notice of acknowledging the voluntary relinquishment and the reason(s) for it, the practitioner shall be given an opportunity to request, within 10 days, a meeting with the credentials committee, the department's EPP, and the chief of staff. During that meeting, the practitioner shall have an opportunity to explain or discuss extenuating circumstances involving his or her failure to provide sufficient clinical experience for a satisfactory evaluation. At that meeting none of the parties shall be represented by counsel, minutes shall be kept, the practitioner may present evidence of extenuating circumstances and why the evaluation period should be extended, any party may ask questions of any party relative to the practitioner's appointment or clinical privileges.

3. At the conclusion of the meeting, the credentials committee shall make a written report and recommendation. The report shall include the minutes of the meeting held with the practitioner. After reviewing the credential's committee recommendation and report, the MEC shall either adopt the credentials committee's recommendation as its own, send the matter back to the credentials committee with specific concerns or questions, or make a recommendation different than the credential's committee outlining specific reasons for disagreement. The decision of the board shall be final.

4. The practitioner shall not be entitled to a hearing or other procedural rights as set forth in the medical staff bylaws or the fair hearing and appeal policy for any privilege that is voluntarily relinquished.

Figure 3.1	Focused professional practice evaluations (cont.)

XI. Procedural rights: Recommendations for termination of appointment or reduction in clinical privileges:

If there is a recommendation by the MEC to terminate the practitioner's appointment or additional clinical privileges due to questions about qualifications, behavior, or clinical competence, the practitioner shall be entitled to the hearing and appeal process outlined in the medical staff bylaws and the fair hearing and appeal policy.

XII. Responsibilities of the MSO and quality improvement department:

1. Send the practitioner being proctored and to the assigned proctor a letter that contains the following information:

    a. A copy of the privilege form of the practitioner being proctored
    b. The name, addresses, and telephone numbers of both the practitioner being proctored and the proctor
    c. A copy of the proctoring policy and procedure
    d. Proctoring forms to be completed by the proctor

2. Develop a mechanism (in coordination with the information services department) for tracking all admissions or procedures performed by the practitioner being proctored.

3. Contact the proctor and practitioner on a monthly basis to ensure that proctoring and chart reviews are being conducted as required. In the absence of receiving proctoring reports, contact the proctor and practitioner.

4. Periodically submit a report to the MEC of proctorship activity for all practitioners being proctored.

5. At the conclusion of the proctoring period, submit a summary proctor report to the credential committee and MEC.

Source: MeritCare Health System, Fargo, ND.

| Figure 3.2 | Departmental policy on focused professional practice evaluations |

Note: *To ensure consistency among the various departments, a template was created to assist each department in developing a department-specific focused professional practice evaluation (FPPE) plan. This is a concept document that presents the framework for specialties to use in the creation of a specialty specific FPPE process.*

It is also important to note that these documents reflect the leadership involvement and commitment to FPPE in this organization. It takes time and clinical expertise to evaluate the scope of practice of a particular specialty and delineate how competence would be demonstrated within that clinical discipline.

The privileging system used by an organization will be the first step in defining how FPPE will be done. Generally, the organization will determine the FPPE plan for a practitioner based upon the way clinical privileges are delineated for that specialty.

Purpose: To establish a departmental proctoring policy that ensures that there is sufficient information available to confirm the competence of a [*fill in the blank*] who initially requests privileges at MeritCare Hospital within the department of [*fill in the blank*]. This policy is not intended to be all encompassing. It outlines the minimum requirements. The credentials committee or departmental members may determine that a practitioner requires more than this minimum to ensure competency and safety.

As per the proctoring policy adopted by the medical staff executive committee of MeritCare Hospital, proctoring includes one or more of the following:

1. Presentation of cases with planned treatment outlined for treatment concurrence or review of case documentation for treatment concurrence (prospective proctoring)

2. Real-time observation of a procedure (concurrent proctoring)

3. Review of a case after care has been completed, which may include interviews with personnel involved in the care of the patient (retrospective proctoring)

4. Evidence of successful proctoring at another local hospital, subject to the requirements noted below (reciprocal observation)

The [*fill in the blank*] department will take into account the practitioner's previous experience in determining the approach and extent of proctoring needed to confirm current competence. The practitioner's experience may fall into one of the following classes:

1. Recent graduate from a training program affiliated with MeritCare Health System, where the requested privileges were part of the training program

2. Recent graduate from a training program at another facility, where the requested privileges were part of the training program

| Figure 3.2 | Departmental policy on focused professional practice evaluations (cont.) |

3. A practitioner with regular experience exercising the requested privilege of fewer than two years on another medical staff

4. A practitioner with regular experience exercising the requested privilege of more than five years at another medical staff

Minimum requirements for class one practitioners:

- No concurrent proctoring required, although the department at its discretion may request it, as the practitioner has been proctored by MeritCare staff through out his or her residency.

- Retrospective review of the practitioners first [*fill in the number*] independently handled admissions/procedures.

Minimum requirements for class two and three practitioners:

- Prospective proctoring of [*fill in the number*] cases

- Concurrent proctoring of [*fill in the number*] procedures, to include:

  - [*consider listing two or three common procedures*]

    Note: This area of concurrent proctoring is applicable only to proceduralists.

- Retrospective review of [*fill in the number*] cases

Minimum requirements for class four practitioners include at least one of the following:

- Evidence of reciprocal observation as described in the medical staff policy on proctoring

- Retrospective review of the practitioner's first [*fill in the number*] admissions

The departmental executive physician partner or managing physician partner will assign the mentor for each new practitioner. He or she is expected to contact the office of physician practice at [*phone number*] and receive the appropriate review materials. Upon completion, they will be returned via mail to the office of physician practice at [*address*] and forwarded to the credentials committee.

Source: MeritCare Health System, Fargo, ND.

| Figure 3.3 | Prospective proctoring: Cognitive diagnostic/Medical evaluation form |

Note: The prospective proctoring for cognitive diagnostic/medical evaluation is best accomplished by an early discussion between the newly privileged applicant and the proctor. A sample scenario would be if a newly privileged family practitioner or internist has just seen a patient in the emergency room presenting with chest pain. The new practitioner would call the proctor, describe the physical findings and laboratory results with the proctor, and outline his or her plans for therapeutic management of this patient (e.g., admission to the intensive care unit for further monitoring or cardiology consult). The proctor would then document the interaction following further evaluation of the patient or patient's chart, as indicated.

Confidential peer review document

To: Chair, department of _____

Date: _____

Confidential for file of: _____
                                                    (Practitioner's name)

Name of proctor: _____

Patient record identifier: _____

Diagnosis: _____

_____

_____

Procedure: _____

_____

_____

Complications: _____

_____

Figure 3.3	Prospective proctoring: Cognitive diagnostic/Medical evaluation form (cont.)

Please answer all of the following.
If the answer to any of the following questions is no, please attach an explanation on a separate sheet.

Yes	No	N/A	
			1. Was there adequate evidence to support the patient's admission?
			2. Was the proposed initial level of care appropriate?
			3. Was the practitioner's problem formulation (e.g., initial impressions, rules outs, assessment, etc.) appropriate?
			4. Did the practitioner cooperate with you concerning this review?
			5. Was all necessary information (e.g., history, physical, progress notes, operative notes, and summary) recorded by the practitioner in a timely manner in the patient's medical record?
			6. Was the above information recorded legibly?
			7. Were the entries made in the patient's record by the practitioner informative?
			8. Were the entries made in the patient's record by the practitioner appropriate?
			9. Was the practitioner's proposed use of diagnostic services (e.g., lab, x-ray, and invasive diagnostic procedures) appropriate?
			10. Were the practitioner's proposed initial orders appropriate?
			11. Was the practitioner's proposed drug use appropriate?
			12. Was the practitioner's proposed use of blood and blood components appropriate?
			13. Was the practitioner's proposed use of ancillary services (physical therapy, respiratory therapy, social service, etc.) appropriate?

Basic Assessment	Satisfactory	Unsatisfactory
1. Basic medical knowledge		
2. Clinical judgment		
3. Communication skills		
4. Use of consultants		
5. Professional attitude		
6. Recordkeeping		
7. Relationship to patient		

Generally, how would you rate this practitioner's skill and competence in performing this examination?

❑ Outstanding ❑ Acceptable ❑ Unacceptable
❑ Unable to evaluate because: _____

_____
_____

General comments: _____

_____
_____

Source: MeritCare Health System, Fargo, ND.

Figure 3.4	Concurrent proctoring: Cognitive diagnostic/medical evaluation form

Confidential peer review document

To: Chair, department of _____

Date: _____

Confidential for file of: _____
(Practitioner's name)

Name of proctor: _____

Patient record identifier: _____

Diagnosis: _____
_____
_____

Procedure: _____
_____
_____

Complications: _____
_____
_____

Please answer all of the following. If the answer to any of the following questions (except for questions 18 and 19, where a yes answer requires explanation) is no, please attach an explanation on a separate sheet.

Yes	No	N/A	Diagnostic work-up
			1. Was there adequate evidence to support the patient's admission?
			2. Was the initial level of care appropriate?
			3. Was the practitioner's problem formulation (e.g., initial impressions, rules-outs, assessment, etc.) appropriate?
			4. Were patient rounds made daily?
			5. Did the practitioner cooperate with you concerning this review?
			6. Did the practitioner record all necessary information (e.g., history, physical, progress notes, operative notes, and summary) in a timely manner in the patient's medical record?
			7. Was the above information recorded in a legible manner?

Figure 3.4	Concurrent proctoring: Cognitive diagnostic/medical evaluation form (cont.)

			8. Were the entries made in the patient's record by the practitioner informative?
			9. Were the entries made in the patient's record by the practitioner appropriate?
			10. Was the practitioner's proposed use of diagnostic services (e.g., lab, x-ray, and invasive diagnostic procedures) appropriate?
			11. Were the practitioner's initial orders appropriate?

Yes	No	N/A	Patient management
			12. Was the practitioner's drug use appropriate?
			13. Was the practitioner's use of blood and blood components appropriate?
			14. Was the practitioner's use of ancillary services (e.g., physical therapy, respiratory therapy, social service, etc.) appropriate?
			15. Were complications anticipated, recognized promptly, and dealt with appropriately?
			16. Was the patient's length of stay appropriate?

Yes	No	N/A	Patient discharge
			17. Was the patient discharged to an appropriate level of care?

Yes	No	N/A	Relationship with patients and hospital employees
			18. Was there any evidence that the practitioner exhibited any disruptive or inappropriate behavior?
			19. Was there any evidence of patient dissatisfaction with the practitioner?

Basic Assessment	Satisfactory	Unsatisfactory
1. Basic medical knowledge		
2. Clinical judgment		
3. Communication skills		
4. Use of consultants		
5. Professional attitude		
6. Recordkeeping		
7. Relationship to patient		

Generally, how would you rate this practitioner's skill and competence in performing this examination?

❏ Outstanding ❏ Acceptable ❏ Unacceptable
❏ Unable to evaluate because: _____

_____
_____

General comments: _____

_____
_____

Source: MeritCare Health System, Fargo, ND.

| Figure 3.5 | Prospective proctoring procedural/surgical evaluation form |

Note: The prospective proctoring for procedural/surgical evaluation would be accomplished through a preprocedure conversation with the newly privileged practitioner and the proctor. A sample scenario would be if a newly privileged general surgeon evaluated a patient in the emergency room and had a preoperative diagnosis of a bowel obstruction necessitating the patient being taken to the operating room. The new practitioner would call the proctor, describe the findings to him or her, and outline the surgical management of the case. The proctor would then document the interaction following further evaluation of the patient or patient's chart as indicated.

Confidential peer review document

To: Chair, department of _____

Date: _____

Confidential for file of: _____

(Practitioner's name)

Name of proctor: _____

Patient record identifier: _____

Diagnosis: _____

_____

_____

Procedure: _____

_____

_____

Complications: _____

_____

Figure 3.5	Prospective proctoring procedural/surgical evaluation form (cont.)

Please answer all of the following. If the answer to any of the following questions is no, please attach an explanation on a separate sheet.

Yes	No	N/A		
			1.	Was there preoperative justification for the proposed surgery?
			2.	Did the practitioner record all necessary information (e.g., history, physical, progress notes, operative notes, and summary) in a timely manner in the patient's medical record?
			3.	Was the above information recorded legibly?
			4.	Were the entries made in the patient's record by the practitioner informative?
			5.	Were the entries made in the patient's record by the practitioner appropriate?
			6.	Was the practitioner's use of diagnostic services (e.g., lab, x-ray, and invasive diagnostic procedures) appropriate?
			7.	Was the practitioner's proposed surgical technique appropriate?
			8.	Were the practitioner's contingency plans appropriate?

Basic Assessment	Satisfactory	Unsatisfactory
1. Basic medical knowledge		
2. Clinical judgment		
3. Communication skills		
4. Use of consultants		
5. Professional attitude		
6. Recordkeeping		
7. Relationship to patient		

Generally, how would you rate this practitioner's skill and competence in performing this examination?

❏ Outstanding ❏ Acceptable ❏ Unacceptable
❏ Unable to evaluate because: _____
_____
_____

General comments: _____
_____
_____

Source: MeritCare Health System, Fargo, ND.

| Figure 3.6 | Concurrent proctoring: Procedural/surgical evaluation form |

Confidential peer review document

To: Chair, department of _____

Date: _____

Confidential for file of: _____

(Practitioner's name)

Name of proctor: _____

Patient record identifier: _____

Diagnosis: _____

_____

_____

Procedure: _____

_____

_____

Complications: _____

_____

_____

Figure 3.6	Concurrent proctoring: Procedural/surgical evaluation form (cont.)

Please answer all of the following. If the answer to any of the following questions (except for questions 15 and 16, where a yes answer requires explanation) is no, please attach an explanation on a separate sheet.

Yes	No	N/A	
			1. Was there preoperative justification for the surgery documented?
			2. Were patient rounds made daily?
			3. Did the practitioner answer calls promptly?
			4. Did the practitioner cooperate with you concerning this review?
			5. Was all necessary information (e.g., history, physical, progress notes, operative notes, and summary) recorded by the practitioner in a timely manner in the patient's medical record?
			6. Was the above information recorded legibly?
			7. Were the entries made in the patient's record by the practitioner informative?
			8. Were the entries made in the patient's record by the practitioner appropriate?
			9. Was the practitioner's use of diagnostic services (e.g., lab, x-ray, and invasive diagnostic procedures) appropriate?
			10. Was the practitioner's surgical technique appropriate?
			11. Did the preoperative diagnosis coincide with postoperative findings?
			12. Was postoperative care adequate?
			13. Was the operative report complete, accurate, and timely?
			14. Were complications, if any, recognized and managed appropriately?
			15. Was there any evidence that the practitioner exhibited any disruptive or inappropriate behavior?
			16. Was there any evidence of patient dissatisfaction with the practitioner?

Generally, how would you rate this practitioner's skill and competence in performing this examination?

❏ Outstanding   ❏ Acceptable   ❏ Unacceptable
❏ Unable to evaluate because: _____
_____
_____

General comments: _____
_____
_____

Source: MeritCare Health System, Fargo, ND.

Figure 3.7	Retrospective proctoring: Case rating form

Medical record number: _____

Discharge date: _____

Provider number: _____ Department: _____

Diagnosis: _____

Procedure/surgery (if applicable): _____

Case summary _____

To be completed by physician reviewer

Physician reviewer: _____

Review date: _____

Circle worst condition that applies for outcome and effect on patient care (independent of physician care)

	Outcome
1.	No adverse outcome
2.	Minor adverse outcome (complete recovery expected)
3.	Major adverse outcome (complete recovery not expected)
4.	Death

	Effect of patient care
1.	Care not affected
2.	Increased level of monitoring/observation (e.g., vital sign checks)
3.	Additional treatment/intervention (e.g., IV fluids)
4.	Life-sustaining treatment/intervention (e.g., intubation, pressor support, CPR, prolonged length of stay)

	Documentation: Circle all that apply
A.	No issue with documentation
B.	Documentation not present
C.	Documentation does not substantiate clinical course and treatment
D.	Documentation not timely to communicate with other caregivers
E.	Documentation illegible
F.	Other:

Figure 3.7	Retrospective proctoring: Case rating form (cont.)

Note regarding the following two tables: If issue A is identified, then overall care selected must be 1. If one of issues B through H is selected, then the overall care selected must be 2 or 3.

	Issue identification
A.	No issues with physician care identified
B.	Diagnosis
C.	Judgment
D.	Technique/skill
E.	Communication or implementation of treatment plan
F.	Policy compliance
G.	Supervision of allied health practitioner/house staff
H.	Other:

	Overall physician care: Circle one
1.	Care appropriate
2.	Care unusual or questionable
3.	Care inappropriate

If overall physician care rated 2 or 3, please provide brief description of the following:

Basis for reviewer findings: _____

Exemplary nominations:

_____ Overall care exemplary   _____ Documentation exemplary

Brief description: _____
_____
_____

Source: MeritCare Health System, Fargo, ND.

Figure 3.8	Ongoing physician feedback policy

Note: *As part of focused professional practice evaluation (FPPE) and the ongoing professional practice evaluation (OPPE), MeritCare uses physician feedback reports. An element of interest in this document is the definitions created to evaluate care provided.*

Purpose: To establish an objective, systematic process to ensure that there is sufficient evidence-based information relevant to the clinical activity of each member of the medical staff and each advanced practice professional staff member. These activities comprise the majority of the functions of the ongoing peer review process. The data is used as part of the reappointment process and decisions to maintain existing privileges to revise existing privileges or to revoke such privileges.

Definitions: Medical/professional staff members will have ongoing department-/specialty-specific feedback in the following areas:

- Clinical/technical quality: This refers to a medical/professional staff member's clinical skills. The medical staff and each department establish expectations regarding such skill, and these expectations address patient outcomes and specific clinical processes. Some of these processes may be common to the entire medical staff. For example, all physicians are expected to provide for patient comfort.

- Service quality: This refers to a medical/professional staff member's accessibility and focus on patient satisfaction. This includes patient and coworker complaints regarding behavioral issues.

- Patient safety: This addresses how a medical/professional staff member's care ensures safe practices and respect for patient safety—for example, by including the date and time of orders.

- Resource utilization: This addresses the fact that resources are finite and that all practitioners must share these limited resources in ways that maximize care for the greatest number of patients.

- Citizenship: This refers to the fact that being a member of the medical/professional staff is a privilege, not a right, and with that comes responsibilities. These may include attending meetings, participating in quality improvement activities, and cooperating with peer review work. It answers the question, "What do we expect of each other?"

Scope: This policy applies to all medical staff members with privileges and advanced practice professional staff members with privileges. The feedback reports are to be reviewed either quarterly or at a minimum twice a year by the medical/professional staff member and his or her executive physician partner or managing physician partner (MPP). Portions may be used at the time of reappointment as determined by departmental policy, as approved by the executive committee and the board of directors.

| Figure 3.8 | Ongoing physician feedback policy (cont.) |

Procedure:

A. **Responsibilities of credentials committee, MPPs, executive physician partners (EPP), and departments:** The medical staff committees or departments involved with OPPE will provide the credentials committee with evidenced-based information regarding clinical activity that is systematically collected through the OPPE processes for appropriate members of the medical/professional staff. MPPs and EPPs are responsible for working with their departments to annually review and improve the performance feedback reports, as well as working with individual medical/professional staff members within their department to improve performance. Each department will determine the threshold for acceptable and excellent performance for those indicators that are department specific, subject to approval of the executive committee and board of directors. The board of directors of the hospital may, at its discretion and after consultation with the executive committee, establish a hospital or system indicator, which will set the performance expectations.

B. **Method:** Each clinical department will be responsible for developing indicators and performance thresholds specific to that department for each of the categories listed above, subject to approval of the executive committee and the board of directors. These should be reviewed on an annual basis. Where possible, indicators will be those that provide an opportunity for medical/professional staff member–specific feedback of data. The medical staff executive committee will establish and annually review hospitalwide indicator(s) and performance expectations that will be pertinent to all departments (e.g., noting date and time of orders), subject to approval of the board of directors.

The clinical departments, in conjunction with the quality improvement department, will conduct performance measurement and construction of the feedback reports based on identified areas of opportunity for improvement. Frequency of feedback reporting will also be determined at the department and provider level, but no less than twice per year.

The quality improvement department will populate and distribute all feedback reports. Analysis of performance will occur at the individual department level. For those indicators that are hospitalwide, the analysis will also be reported to the executive committee and to the quality committee of the board of directors on a quarterly basis, where applicable.

C. **Consequences of poor performance:** Medical/professional staff members who are found to be at less than the hospital's or department's established threshold for performance will be required to develop a plan for improvement in conjunction with their department's MPP or clinical EPP.

If the medical/professional staff member performs below threshold expectations, the MPP or EPP may recommend/require an FPPE. Please see that policy for details.

Figure 3.8	Ongoing physician feedback policy (cont.)

D. **Responsibilities of EPPs or MPPs:**

The EPP (or MPP when there is no EPP for the department, is expected to:)

1. Facilitate the annual review of departmental indicators
2. Annually meet with each medical/professional staff member in his or her areas of responsibility to review his or her performance and provide personal feedback
3. Review each medical/professional staff member's performance and, when needed, develop improvement plans that address any identified deficiencies or areas for improvement
4. Request, when needed, an FPPE

E. **Responsibilities of the medical staff office and quality improvement (QI) department:**

1. The medical staff office will receive a copy of each medical/professional staff member's quarterly or semiannual report and will place that in the quality section of his or her credentials file. This will be available to the credentials committee, chief-of-staff, EPP, and MPP of the medical/professional staff member's department.
2. The QI department will be responsible for populating and distributing all templates to the individual medical/professional staff members and their EPP or MPP.
3. The QI department will be responsible for working with each department on an annual basis to review the continued relevance of the indicators chosen and will assist with updating the indicators as directed by the department.

Source: MeritCare Health System, Fargo, ND.

Figure 3.9	Anesthesia: Focused professional physician evaluation plan

Refer to the MeritCare Health System Proctoring policy for initially requested privileges (Figure 3.1) for background, definitions, and specific responsibilities of the proctors and managing physician partner (MPP).

Proctoring methods: The anesthesia department will utilize primarily concurrent proctoring and retrospective proctoring. In rare cases, reciprocal proctoring may be used.

Duration and scope of proctoring: Physicians in class two and three will receive full proctoring for such a time as needed to complete the following required observations and reviews:

- Observation of five central line placements, at least one of which should be a subclavian approach

- Observation of three epidural catheter placements, at least one of which should be a thoracic epidural

- Observation of use of advanced airway management modalities at least once each, including Fast-track LMA, Glide Scope, and fiberoptic video bronchoscope

- Observation of one each of a femoral nerve block, interscalene block, and axillary block

- Review of the preoperative evaluation, anesthetic plan, and anesthetic course (from the anesthesia record) of at least three cardiac cases, including one valve, one off-pump coronary artery bypass graft (CABG), and one on-pump CABG

- Review of the preoperative evaluation, anesthetic plan, and anesthetic course (from the anesthesia record) of two pediatric cases and two adult cases for general, ear-nose-throat, urologic, orthopedic, or gynecologic surgery

Physicians in class four will receive minimal proctoring unless there are specific concerns about the physician's recent experience with any of the requested privileges. Minimal proctoring will consist of:

- Observation of use of advanced airway management modalities at least once each, including Fast-track LMA, Glide Scope, and fiberoptic video bronchoscope

- Observation of one each of a femoral nerve block, interscalene block, and axillary block

- Review of the preoperative evaluation, anesthetic plan, and anesthetic course (from the anesthesia record) of at least two cardiac cases of any type

Assignment of proctors: The department MPP will be responsible to assign a proctor to each new physician in the department. It is the responsibility of all department physicians to serve as proctors when asked to do so.

Documentation: The proctors will complete and deliver the proctoring forms to the MeritCare Hospital medical staff office. These forms should be kept confidential. A summary report will also be submitted at the conclusion of the proctoring period.

Source: MeritCare Health System, Fargo, ND.

| Figure 3.10 | Anesthesia: Focused professional physician evaluation plan for CRNA |

> **Note:** *This form contains distinctions between minimal and full proctoring because consideration has been given to the on-site knowledge of practitioners from the formal training program, and therefore the focused professional practice evaluation (FPPE) requirement has been reduced.*

Refer to the MeritCare Health System Proctoring policy for initially requested privileges (Figure 3.1) for background, definitions, and specific responsibilities of the proctors and managing physician partner (MPP).

Proctoring methods: The anesthesia department will utilize prospective, concurrent, and retrospective proctoring. In rare cases, reciprocal proctoring may be used. The certified registered nurse anesthetist (CRNA) will complete the anesthesia department orientation for both North and South Campus departments. This orientation will be used in conjunction with the FPPE plan for the CRNA to complete all proctoring requirements.

Duration and scope of proctoring: The CRNA with previous clinical experience or those who performed clinical rotations at MeritCare under the University of North Dakota nurse anesthesia program may be eligible for minimal proctoring unless there are specific concerns about the CRNA's recent experience with any of the requested privileges. Minimal proctoring will consist of:

- Review of the preoperative evaluation, anesthetic plan, and anesthetic management (from the anesthesia record) of two neonatal procedures and two cardiac cases of any type

- Observation of use of advanced airway management modalities at least once each, including the C-Trach laryngeal mask airway the MacGrath laryngoscope, the Glide Scope, and fiberoptic video laryngoscope

- Observation of one each of a single-shot femoral nerve block, a continuous femoral nerve block, an interscalene block, and an axillary block

The CRNA will receive full proctoring for such a time as needed to complete the following required observations and reviews:

- Review of the preoperative evaluation, anesthetic plan, and anesthetic management (from the anesthesia record) of at least three cardiac cases, including one valve, one off-pump coronary artery bypass graft (CABG), and one on-pump CABG

- Review of the preoperative evaluation, anesthetic plan, and anesthetic management (from the anesthesia record) of two neonatal cases, two pediatric cases, and two adult cases for general, ear-nose-throat, urologic, orthopedic, neuro, plastic, or gynecologic surgical procedures

- Review of the preoperative evaluation, anesthetic plan, and anesthetic management of two nonsurgical procedures—that is, electroconvulsive therapy, magnetic resonance imaging, and computerized axial tomography scans; pediatric bone marrow biopsies; intrathecal chemo injections, endoscopic or transesophageal echocardiogram procedures; radiologic procedures; and cath lab procedures

Figure 3.10	Anesthesia: Focused professional physician evaluation plan for CRNA (cont.)

- Observation of the use of advanced airway management modalities at least once for each of the following: the MacGrath laryngoscope, the C-Trach LMA, the Glide Scope, and fiber-optic video laryngoscope (note observation will also include the administration of airway blocks utilized for awake intubations)

- Observation of one each: a single-shot femoral nerve block, a continuous femoral nerve block, an interscalene block, and an axillary block

- Observation of an epidural catheter placement

A CRNA requesting privileges to perform epidural blocks will make arrangements with the proctor to observe the placement of ten epidural catheters. A documentation record of these blocks will be maintained in the anesthesia department.

A CRNA requesting privileges to perform the following blocks: interscalene blocks, axillary block, femoral nerve blocks, and continuous femoral nerve blocks will be required to make arrangements with the proctor to perform 10 supervised blocks of each type of block for which privileges are requested. A documentation record of these blocks will be maintained in the anesthesia department. The CRNA will complete the requirements to obtain privileges for one type of block at a time.

Assignment of proctors: The manager or lead CRNAs will assign proctors to each new CRNA in the department. It is the responsibility of all department CRNAs to serve as proctors when asked to do so.

Documentation: The proctors will complete and deliver the proctoring forms to the MeritCare Hospital medical staff office. The forms to be completed will include:

1. Retrospective proctoring, case rating form; minimum two

2. Concurrent proctoring, procedural/surgical evaluation form; minimum three, including one cardiovascular procedure, one adult general surgery procedure, and one pediatric diagnostic or surgical procedure

The proctor will ensure the confidentiality of the forms. A summary report will also be submitted at the conclusion of the proctoring period.

Source: MeritCare Health System, Fargo, ND.

| Figure 3.11 | Critical care medicine: Proctoring policy |

Note: This specialty has determined that the newly privileged practitioner will spend a minimum of five days in orientation and being observed to confirm clinical and procedural skills prior to being allowed to take independent call.

Purpose: To ensure clinical and procedural competence for new physicians in the MeritCare critical care medicine department. This policy applies to permanent and temporary physicians.

Policy: A period of orientation to the critical care department will occur for every new physician joining the critical care department. The duration of this orientation will be a minimum of five days and can be extended if deemed necessary. The orientation will be done by one or several of the current physician members of the MeritCare critical care department as assigned by the managing physician partner (MPP) of critical care services.

The orientation will include but is not limited to participation in critical care teaching rounds, confirmation of clinical skills (allowing the new physician to manage a limited number of patients with immediate back-up as needed), confirmation of procedural skills (allowing the new physician to do procedures with immediate back-up as needed), and meetings with the key departments that form the core critical care team. The specific duties and tasks to be accomplished during the orientation will be determined by the proctor and the MPP.

The new physician will not be allowed to take independent call for the critical care service until successful completion of the orientation. The physician will receive a letter from the MPP upon successful completion of the orientation.

Source: MeritCare Health System, Fargo, ND.

| Figure 3.12 | Emergency: Focused professional physician evaluation plan |

Evaluation and management: Physician candidates new to MeritCare's emergency department will have five patient encounters observed by a proctor prior to independent practice within the department. This should occur within the first three days of arrival and must occur within one week. If any concern arises regarding a candidate's performance, it will immediately be reported to [*fill in the blank*] and an additional 10 encounters will be observed and further action taken as recommended by [*fill in the blank*].

In addition to the observation of real-time patient encounters, the proctor will review and assess the evaluation and management documented in the medical record for 25 patient encounters. If any concern exists regarding a candidate's performance as documented in the medical record, it will immediately be reported to [*fill in the blank*], and an additional 50 records will be reviewed with further action taken as recommended by [*fill in the blank*].

Procedural: Physicians new to MeritCare and MeritCare's emergency department will have two of each of the following procedures observed, and documentation for the same, reviewed prior to independently performing the procedures within the department:

1. Laceration repair and wound management

2. Orthopedic splinting and injury management

3. Epistaxis management

4. Corneal foreign body removal and management

5. Lumbar puncture

6. Abscess incision and drainage, and subsequent management

7. Endotracheal intubation

In addition to these procedures, physicians performing less common but high-risk procedures, including central venous lines, arterial lines, chest tube thoracostomy, thoracentesis, and para-centesis, should have the first procedure performed within the department observed and the documentation for the same procedure reviewed.

Assurance of continuous quality of care: Any concerns voiced on the part of emergency department or other hospital staff (e.g., physicians, nurses, administrators) following the initial proctoring period will be considered on a case-by-case basis. If the concern relates to quality of patient care and is with merit, it will be immediately reported to [*fill in the blank*] and further action taken as recommended by [*fill in the blank*] in consultation with the emergency department managing physician partner.

Source: MeritCare Health System, Fargo, ND.

| Figure 3.13 | Pediatrics: Focused professional physician evaluation plan |

Purpose: To establish a departmental proctoring policy that ensures that sufficient information is available to confirm the competence of a pediatrician or pediatric subspecialist who initially requests privileges at MeritCare Children's Hospital. This policy is not intended to be all encompassing. It outlines the minimum requirements. The credentials committee or departmental members may determine that a practitioner requires more than this minimum to ensure competency and safety.

As per the proctoring policy adopted by the medical staff executive committee of MeritCare Hospital, proctoring includes one or more of the following:

> **Note:** This specialty has incorporated prospective, concurrent, and retrospective review into its focused professional practice evaluation plan.

1. Presentation of a minimum of five cases with planned treatment outlined for treatment concurrence or review of case documentation for treatment concurrence

2. Real-time observation of procedures such as circumcision, intubation, central line placement, etc.

3. Review of a minimum of five cases after care has been completed, which will include interviews with personnel involved in the care of the patient

4. Evidence of successful proctoring at another local hospital, subject to the requirements noted below

MeritCare Children's Hospital will take into account the practitioner's previous experience in determining the approach and extent of proctoring needed to confirm current competence. The practitioner's experience may fall into one of the following classes:

1. Recent graduate from a training program affiliated with MeritCare Health System, where the requested privileges were part of the training program

2. Recent graduate from a training program at another facility, where the requested privileges were part of the training program

3. A practitioner with regular experience exercising the requested privilege of fewer than five years on another medical staff

4. A practitioner with regular experience exercising the requested privilege of more than five years at another medical staff

Figure 3.13	Pediatrics: Focused professional physician evaluation plan (cont.)

Minimum requirements for class one practitioners:

- No concurrent proctoring required, although the department may, at its discretion, request it, as the practitioner has been proctored by MeritCare staff through out his or her residency

- Retrospective review of the practitioner's first five independently handled admissions or procedures

Minimum requirements for class two and three practitioners:

- Prospective proctoring of a minimum of five cases

- Concurrent proctoring of a minimum of five procedures, to include:

    - Procedures germane to the division, such as circumcision, central line placement, intubation, etc.

Note: This area of concurrent proctoring is applicable only to proceduralists:

- Retrospective review of a minimum of five cases.

Minimum requirements for class four practitioners include any of the following:

- Evidence of reciprocal observation as described in the medical staff policy on proctoring

- Retrospective review of the practitioner's first five admissions

- The departmental executive physician partner or managing physician partner will assign the mentor for each new practitioner. He or she is expected to contact the office of physician practice at [phone number] and receive the appropriate review materials. Upon completion, the materials will be returned to the office of physician practice at [mailing address] and forwarded to the credentials committee.

Source: MeritCare Health System, Fargo, ND.

| Figure 3.14 | Psychiatry: Focused professional physician evaluation plan |

This document is to be used in conjunction with the MeritCare Health System proctoring policy for initially requested privileges (Figure 3.1).

The medical staff will take into account the practitioner's previous experience in determining the approach and extent of proctoring needed to confirm current competence. The practitioner's experience may fall into one of the following classes:

1. Recent graduate from a training program affiliated with MeritCare Health System, where the requested privileges were part of the training program

2. Recent graduate from training program at another facility, where the requested privileges were part of the training program

3. A practitioner with regular experience exercising the requested privileges with fewer than three years on another medical staff

4. A practitioner with regular experience exercising the requested privilege with more than three years on another medical staff

Minimal expectations for proctoring of each class of practitioner are outlined below. Extent of proctoring will be determined individually, and the department may elect at its discretion to require more than the minimum expectation.

- Practitioners in class one will need no proctoring, because MeritCare has had the opportunity to observe the current competence of the applicant directly.

- Practitioners in classes two, three, and four will have full proctoring, as defined below.

Proctoring definitions are as follows: The proctor's role is that of an evaluator—to review and observe cases—not of a supervisor or consultant. The practitioner who is serving solely as a proctor is an agent of the hospital. The proctor receives no compensation directly or indirectly from any patient for this service.

1. Proctors must be members in good standing of the active medical staff of MeritCare Hospital and must have unrestricted privileges to perform any procedure(s) to be concurrently proctored.

2. Proctors shall directly observe the patient interview or procedure being performed and concurrently proctor medical management for the medical admission and complete appropriate sections of the proctoring form.

3. Proctors will retrospectively review the completed medical record following discharge and complete appropriate sections of the proctoring form.

| Figure 3.14 | Psychiatry: Focused professional physician evaluation plan (cont.) |

This plan exemplifies focused professional practice evaluation for a nonprocedural specialty.

4. The proctor will monitor the practitioner being proctored from admission to discharge, including the following, as applicable to the patient and standard psychiatric practice:

- History and physical
- Diagnosis and justification of same
- Proposed treatment or procedure and its indications
- Continuity of care provided to the patients
- Appropriateness of tests, procedures, and medications prescribed
- Appropriate use of consultants
- Appropriateness of length of stay
- Adequacy and legibility of progress notes
- Discharge summary
- Timely completion of medical records
- Appropriately signed consents
- Technical skills/knowledge (as appropriate)
- Management of complications

5. Full proctoring requirements will include these outlined steps for three complete hospital admissions

6. Proctoring for the procedure of electroconvulsive therapy (ECT) will entail the following for a total of three cases:

- Prospective discussion of indication for treatment, planned approach, potential complications and prevention, expected outcomes, etc.
- Concurrent observation of procedure during the ECT series
- Retrospective review of case documentation and outcome after case is completed

Source: MeritCare Health System, Fargo, ND.

| Figure 3.15 | Urology: Focused professional physician evaluation plan |

Purpose: To establish a departmental proctoring policy that ensures that there is sufficient information available to confirm the competence of a urologist who initially requests privileges at MeritCare Hospital within the department of urology. This policy is not intended to be all encompassing. It outlines the minimum requirements. The credentials committee or departmental members may determine that a practitioner requires more than this minimum to ensure competency and safety.

As per the proctoring policy adopted by the medical staff executive committee of MeritCare Hospital, proctoring includes one or more of the following:

- Presentation of cases with planned treatment outlined for treatment concurrence or review of case documentation for treatment concurrence (prospective proctoring)

- Real-time observation of a procedure (concurrent proctoring)

- Review of a case after care has been completed, which may include interviews with personnel involved in the care of the patient (retrospective proctoring)

- Evidence of successful proctoring at another local hospital, subject to the requirements noted below (reciprocal observation)

The department of urology will take into account the practitioner's previous experience in determining the approach and extent of proctoring needed to confirm current competence. The practitioner's experience may fall into one of the following classes:

- Recent graduate from a training program affiliated with MeritCare Health System, where the requested privileges were part of the training program

- Recent graduate from a training program at another facility, where the requested privileges were part of the training program

- A practitioner with regular experience exercising the requested privilege, with fewer than two years on another medical staff

- A practitioner with regular experience exercising the requested privilege, with more than five years at another medical staff

Minimum requirements for class one practitioners: Not applicable, as MeritCare does not have a urologic surgery residency.

Minimum requirements for class two and three practitioners:

- Prospective proctoring of zero cases

- Concurrent proctoring of six procedures, to include three open and three endoscopic cases

| Figure 3.15 | Urology: Focused professional physician evaluation plan (cont.) |

Note: This area of concurrent proctoring is applicable only to proceduralists.

- Retrospective review of three cases

Minimum requirements for class four practitioners:

- Evidence of reciprocal observation as described in the medical staff policy on proctoring
- Retrospective review of the practitioner's first admission
- Concurrent proctoring of one open case and one endoscopic case

The departmental executive physician partner or managing physician partner will assign the proctor for each new practitioner. He or she is expected to contact the office of physician practice at [*phone number*] and receive the appropriate review materials. Upon completion, the materials will be returned to the office of physician practice at [*mailing address*] and forwarded to the credentials committee.

Source: MeritCare Health System, Fargo, ND.

St. John's Health System, Springfield, MO

St. John's Health System is an integrated health system that features a level-one trauma center and is ranked as the third most integrated health system in the nation. The organization has 950 beds and a 673-member medical staff at its main hospital, and it recently expanded its facilities. Since 2003, St. John's moved forward with an ambitious $340 million master plan that included the development of an ambulatory surgery center and medical office building, a new emergency room, new outpatient imaging, new surgical and cardiac intensive care units, and a new energy center on the main campus. The organization is accredited by The Joint Commission (formerly JCAHO), NCQA, the Commission on Accreditation of Rehabilitation Facilities, Accreditation Association for Ambulatory Health Care, and URAC (formerly Utilization Review Accreditation Commission).

Diane Meldi, MBA, CPMSM, CPCS, administrator of medical staff services at St. John's Health System, had an active role in the development of her organization's focused professional practice evaluation (FPPE), which included revising existing procedures and policies, as well as creating new forms. It took the organization a total of nine months to develop, approve, and implement its FPPE policy. Originally, the medical staff office (MSO) intended for the medical staff to take the lead on this project, but finally it was the MSO that drove the process with active involvement by the medical staff.

One obstacle that the organization faced in developing its new FPPE policies and procedures was selecting a reporting format and data collection process that best fit its needs. To overcome this obstacle, the organization budgeted for a full-time employee who was responsible for proctoring and ongoing monitoring projects.

Figure 4.1	Monitoring and peer review policy

Note: As mentioned in the profile at the beginning of this chapter, this health system is highly integrated. Approximately 72% of the medical staff members at St. John's Hospital in Springfield are employees of the health system. Therefore, St. John's policies and procedures, processes, and forms reflect a broad evaluation of the care provided. At St. John's, the system encompasses the full continuum of care—that is, the management of patients in the clinic (practitioner's offices) and the hospital. The scope of the system thus includes ambulatory and acute care, as well as managed care plans. This integration is evident throughout the documents included in this section.

This document is an excerpt from St. John's Health System's complete monitoring and peer review policy. The complete document provides an overview of the entire quality monitoring and peer review process for the system. It is interesting to note the locations of care include multiple hospitals as well as clinic settings. This policy also identifies how initially privileged practitioners will be evaluated (see section IV, policy, items 2–5). Some organizations, like St. John's, separate the focused professional practice evaluation (FPPE) process into a separate policy. Others choose to incorporate FPPE language in the quality improvement plan. Both approaches are acceptable.

I. Purpose: To ensure that St. John's Health System, through the activities of its two medical staffs (St. John's medical staff and St. John's regional medical staff, collectively referred to as medical staff), clinic physicians, and participating practitioners, assesses the performance of individuals granted clinical privileges, practice, or participation and uses the results of such assessments to improve patient care and safety.

II. Goals of monitoring and the peer review process:

1. Improve the quality of care provided by individual practitioners

2. Enhance patient safety

3. Monitor the performance of practitioners who have privileges

4. Identify opportunities for performance improvement

5. Monitor significant trends by analyzing data

6. Ensure that the process for peer review is clearly defined, uniformly investigated, fair, timely, and effective

III. Definitions:

1. Peer review is a process for the evaluation of an individual practitioner's clinical competence and professional conduct and may also include the identification of opportunities to improve patient care. Peer review differs from other quality improvement processes in that it evaluates the strengths and weaknesses of an individual practitioner's performance, rather than appraising the quality of care rendered by a group of professionals or a system.

Figure 4.1	Monitoring and peer review policy (cont.)

Monitoring and peer review is conducted using multiple sources of information, which may include:

- The review of individual cases
- The review of aggregate data for compliance with general rules of the medical staff and clinical standards
- The use of rates in comparison with established benchmarks or norms
- Recognized standards of professional care

Through this process, practitioners receive feedback for personal improvement or confirmation of personal achievement related to the effectiveness of their professional, technical, and inter-personal skills in providing patient care at a St. John's hospital or clinic or with a St. John's health plan.

2. A peer is an individual practicing in the same profession and who has expertise in the appropriate subject matter. The level of subject matter expertise required to provide meaningful evaluation of a practitioner's performance will determine what "practicing in the same profession" means on a case-by-case basis. For example, for quality issues related to general medical care, a physician (MD or DO) may review the care of another practitioner. For specialty-specific clinical issues, such as evaluating the technique of a specialized surgical procedure, a peer is an individual who is well-trained and competent in that surgical specialty.

3. The peer review body reviews findings from the peer review process and assigns the standard of care determination score. The peer review body will assign the practitioner a performance improvement plan, as appropriate. The chair/chief will provide oversight and feedback.

4. A practitioner requested to perform monitoring or peer review may have a conflict of interest in which he or she may not be able to render an unbiased opinion due to either involvement in the patient's care or a relationship with the practitioner involved. It is the obligation of the individual to disclose the potential conflict, and it is the responsibility of the peer review body to determine whether the conflict would prevent the individual from participating and the extent of that participation. Individuals determined to have a conflict may not be present during peer review body discussions or decisions other than to provide information if requested.

IV. Policy:

1. All monitoring and peer review information is privileged and confidential in accordance with the respective medical staff bylaws for St. John's Hospital, St. John's Regional Hospitals, St. John's Clinic, and St. John's Health Plan; state and federal laws; and regulations pertaining to peer review, confidentiality, nondiscoverability, and patient-practitioner privilege.

Figure 4.1	Monitoring and peer review policy (cont.)

2. Practitioners with initially granted privileges without current performance documentation shall be evaluated within 120 days. This evaluation shall be used to assess current clinical competence, practice behavior, and ability to perform requested privileges. (See St. John's Health System Proctoring program for practitioners.)

3. Practitioners with newly granted privileges shall be evaluated as required by privilege criteria or by St. John's Health System Proctoring program for practitioners.

4. The criteria to determine the type of evaluation to be conducted are according to St. John's Health System proctoring program.

5. Medical and surgical proctor's reports shall be used to evaluate performance and clinical competence.

6. Ongoing monitoring of all practitioners shall be according to the performance improvement policy, which shall state specific triggers for focused practitioner review. Ongoing monitoring may include the following:

- Review of operative and other clinical procedure(s) performed and their outcomes

- Pattern of blood and pharmaceutical usage

- Requests for tests and procedures

- Length-of-stay patterns

- Morbidity and mortality data

- Practitioner's use of consultants

- Other relevant criteria as determined by the St. John's Hospital medical executive committee (MEC), clinic executive committee, and the St. John's Regional Hospitals medical staff council (MSC)

The type of data to be collected by St. John's Hospitals and St. John's Clinic is determined by each section chair/clinical service chair/department chair/St. John's Regional Hospitals' medical operating committees and approved by the MEC, clinic executive committee, and MSC.

> Note: St. John's Health System's policy continues past this section. However, for the scope of this book, it is appropriate to end the policy here.

Source: St. John's Health System, Springfield, MO

Figure 4.2	Chart review for peer review/case review referrals

> **Note:** *This form is completed upon referral of a chart for peer review/case review.*

Date assigned: _____ Case review assigned to: _____

Medical record number:	Age:	Patient name:	Sex: ☐ Male ☐ Female	Maxys number:	Discharge date:

Practitioner: _____ Quality review date of letter: _____ Specialty: _____

Department/section: _____ Facility: _____

Date issue identified: _____ Risk manager initials: _____

Source of referral: ☐ Quality ☐ HP   ☐ Patient/staff complaint ☐ Physician/medical staff services   ☐ Risk management ☐ St. John's Clinic

Summary: _____

Complication/injury: _____

Reason for referral:

Date practitioner contacted: _____ | Practitioner comments to be noted below.

General screening

Yes	No	N/A	Check appropriate box for each question
			Is the history and physical adequate to assess the patient's condition and begin the process of diagnosis and treatment?
			Are pre-existing conditions and important risk factors documented?
			Was the diagnosis made in a timely manner?
			Were therapeutic orders and diagnostic tests appropriate?
			If applicable, are the reasons for surgical and/or invasive procedures documented?
			Does the record adequately reflect the clinical course through timely, pertinent progress notes?
			Are handwritten entries legible?

✓	Standard of care/practice recommendation	✓	Outcome of patient care
	Level 1: Managed within standard of care/practice or indeterminate		A: No clinically apparent complication
	Level 2: Minor deviation from standard of care/practice		B: Minor injury—resolved during current hospitalization/treatment
	Level 3: Major deviation from standard of care/practice		C: Moderate injury—prolonged hospitalization/treatment
			D: Major injury—loss of function, permanent injury, death

Figure 4.2	Chart review for peer review/case review referrals (cont.)

Reviewer's conclusion/recommendations:

Issues:	❑ Diagnosis/treatment	❑ Patient non-compliant
	❑ Clinical judgment	❑ Past history of patient's disease
	❑ Clinical technique	❑ System or process issue
	❑ Behavior	❑ Readmission
	❑ Communication	❑ Medication
	❑ Utilization	❑ Delay in diagnosis

Conclusions:	❑ No quality of care concern identified	❑ Further information is needed
	❑ Opportunity for improvement noted	❑ Other

Physician reviewer must contact the practitioner being reviewed to get his/her input regarding peer review case. Comments from practitioner being reviewed: _____

_____
_____
_____

Physician reviewer comments are to be noted on the other side of this document.

Confidential peer review

This material/information has been generated for peer review purposes in accordance with Missouri Peer Review Revised Statute 537.035 and Arkansas Peer Review Statutes 20-9-503 and is considered to be privileged and protected.

MEC/MSC Date:	MEC/MSC Recommendation:

Physician reviewer comments: _____

_____
_____
_____
_____
_____

Source: St. John's Health System, Springfield, MO

| Figure 4.3 | Proctoring program for practitioners |

> *Note:* This program is for practitioners at St. John's Clinic and St. John's Hospitals.

I. Purpose: Clinical proctoring is an important tool for peer review and for evaluating clinical competence of new practitioners seeking privileges or existing practitioners requesting new privileges.

II. Definitions:

A. Proctoring shall mean the concurrent observation of the practitioner's performance of the procedure(s) or treatment by a proctor appointed to so act in accordance with St. John's Clinic and St. John's Hospitals.

B. Monitoring or indirect proctoring shall mean the review and evaluation of a practitioner's performance of a procedure or procedures or patient care generally, principally through review and evaluation by practitioner reviewers of a patient's medical record following performance of the procedure or procedures by the practitioner, or for a specified period of patient care.

C. Executive committee shall mean St. John's Clinic executive committee, St. John's Hospital medical executive committee (MEC), and St. John's Regional Hospitals' medical staff council (MSC).

D. Chief of staff shall mean the applicable St. John's Hospital chief of staff.

E. Department chair shall mean the applicable St. John's Clinic department chair, St. John's Hospital department chair, or St. John's Regional Hospitals' department chair.

F. Section chair shall mean the applicable St. John's Clinic section chair, St. John's Hospital clinical service chair, or St. John's Regional Hospitals' clinical service chair.

III. Procedure for new practitioners requesting privileges:

A. The executive committees will determine which procedures and medical diagnoses shall be required to have practitioner proctoring and monitoring. The section chair/chief of staff will determine two or more high-risk procedures or medical diagnoses that will be proctored. If a specialty does not have a section chair, the department chair/chief of staff will make a recommendation to MEC/MSC regarding the procedures or medical diagnoses to be proctored.

B. Proctoring may be required for new technology, for high-risk procedures, and for any practitioner who is identified and recommended by the credentials committee or medical operating committee and approved by the MEC/MSC.

C. The practitioner being proctored must take the responsibility to arrange the observations. The department chair/chief of staff will be accountable for ensuring that the established practitioners are made available. If no peer specialist is available, the department chair/chief of staff will observe or make arrangements for alternative proctoring. St. John's Health System

Figure 4.3	Proctoring program for practitioners (cont.)

medical staff services shall report to St. John's Clinic and St. John's Hospitals proctoring progress, and the section chair/department chair/chief of staff shall assist with compliance.

D. During the first four months, a practitioner granted privileges for St. John's Clinic, St. John's Hospital, and St. John's Regional Hospitals shall have all proctoring/monitoring completed. All cases must be performed at St. John's clinic or hospital.

E. A proctor shall have the authority to intercede or assist the practitioner when the welfare or safety of a patient is jeopardized by the practitioner being proctored and where it is otherwise appropriate to do so.

F. Proctoring of cases will be completed by practitioners assigned by the section chair, department chair, or chief of staff. Proctors and practitioner reviewers shall hold privileges to perform the procedure or procedures to be proctored or monitored or such other procedures sufficiently similar so that the proctor or practitioner reviewer is sufficiently knowledgeable to be qualified to evaluate the performance of the practitioner. The practitioner reviewer, as applicable, shall be a subspecialist matched as closely as possible to the practitioner's subspecialty or allied health practitioner profession. The proctor shall, upon completion of the observation prepare a written report of the proctor's observations, findings, and evaluation of the practitioner's performance and submit such reports to St. John's Health System medical staff services. Indicators not meeting established criteria will be peer reviewed by the department chair/chief of staff. Any immediate concerns will be handled through the established channels of St. John's Health System peer review policy.

> This is evidence of the impact of the system's integration: St. John's extends its area of responsibility to the practitioner's care provided at other healthcare facilities.

G. St. John's Clinic practitioners who hold privileges in non–St. John's facilities shall abide by the facilities' proctoring requirements. St. John's Clinic practitioners shall forward his or her privilege list of the non–St. John's facility within 90 days of employment to St. John's Health System medical staff services.

H. The department chair/chief of staff will provide a summary report to the executive committee regarding results of the proctoring of the practitioner. A summary report shall also be forwarded to the proctor and the practitioner being proctored. Proctoring reports are not released to the practitioner.

| Figure 4.3 | Proctoring program for practitioners (cont.) |

I. Based on the department chair's/chief of staff's summary report and available quality information, the executive committee will recommend discontinuation, continuation, or modification of the proctoring program for the practitioner. In the event that the executive committee recommends continuation of or modification to the proctoring program, the department chair/chief of staff will provide quarterly updates regarding the progress of the practitioner.

J. If the practitioner is employed with St. John's Clinic, the presidents of the St. John's Clinic will have ultimate accountability for enforcement with St. John's Health System medical staff services' oversight of the documentation of completion and, reporting to appropriate system leadership. To properly evaluate the qualifications of practitioners requesting privileges and to ensure that medical care rendered and surgical procedures performed are of the highest quality, an ongoing and effective proctoring program shall be maintained.

IV. Confidentiality:

A. All minutes, reports, recommendations, communications, and actions made or taken pursuant to this policy are deemed to be covered by the provisions of the Missouri Peer Review Statute, Mo. Ann. Stat. §537.035, as to activities involving St. John's Hospital's Missouri facilities and AR Stat.§20-9-501 and §20-9-503 as to activities involving St. John's Hospital's Arkansas facilities or the corresponding provisions of any subsequent federal or state statute providing protection to peer review or related activities. Further, the committees or panels charged with making reports, findings, recommendations, or investigations pursuant to the policy shall be considered to be acting on behalf of St. John's Hospital(s) and the board(s) when engaged in such professional review activities and thus shall be deemed to be "professional review bodies," as that term is defined in the Health Care Quality Improvement Act of 1986.

It is important to designate where focused professional practice evaluation forms will be filed. Part of this process would be to determine whether protections under state statutes would dictate where these documents should be kept.

B. The original proctoring report shall be filed in the individual practitioner's peer review file.

V. Appeal:

A. Appeal of the decision concerning privileges may be made to the executive committee as provided in the St. John's Hospital(s) medical staff bylaws or St. John's Clinic physicians handbook.

Figure 4.3	Proctoring program for practitioners (cont.)

Proctor's report: Medical or admission

Type of review: ❑ Direct/concurrent review
❑ Monitoring review

Practitioner: _____

Privilege: _____

Proctor: _____

Diagnosis: _____ _____

Date review took place: _____

Medical record number: _____

This proctoring report is confidential and peer review protected. You have been asked to proctor/monitor this practitioner to evaluate the quality of care provided. As such, it is your responsibility to report any poor or significant substandard performance made by the practitioner immediately to the department chair/chief of staff. Please complete the information below and submit this form to the administrator of St. John's Health System medical staff services within 30 days via confidential fax [*fax number*].

Please rate the following elements. Additional sheets may be attached if further space is needed.

Element	Satisfactory	Needs improvment	Unsatisfactory	No information or N/A
Medical knowledge				
Basic medical/clinical knowledge				
Clinical judgment				
Basic clinical judgment				
Quality/appropriateness of patient care outcomes				
Appropriate and timely use of consultants/referrals				
Availability and thoroughness of patient care				
Appropriateness of resource use (admissions, procedures, length of stay, lab, x-ray, tests, etc.)				
Clinical pertinence and completeness of medical records documentation (e.g., history and physical completion)				
Medication and therapeutic regimens appropriate				
Abnormal lab results recognized/followed up				
Case management is consistent with the problem				

| Figure 4.3 | Proctoring program for practitioners (cont.) |

Interpersonal skills				
Ability to work with members of healthcare team				
Rapport with patients and family members				
Communication skills				
Overall communication skills				
Verbal and written fluency in English				
Clarity/legibility of records				
Responsiveness to patient needs				
Demonstrates compassion and palliative care at end of life				
Professionalism				
Timely documentation of medical records				
Plans for follow-up are documented				
Demonstration of ethical standards in treatment				
Maintenance of patient confidentiality				
System-based practice				
Abides by facility medication use policies				
Utilization of clinical practice guidelines				
Abides by facility operations policies				

Comments: _____

_____

_____

_____

Is there any aspect of this evaluation and treatment with which you are uneasy or uncomfortable (marginal or unacceptable evaluations)? _____

_____

Proctor signature: _____

Print name: _____

Date: _____

Source: St. John's Health System, Springfield, MO

Figure 4.4 — Proctoring program algorithm

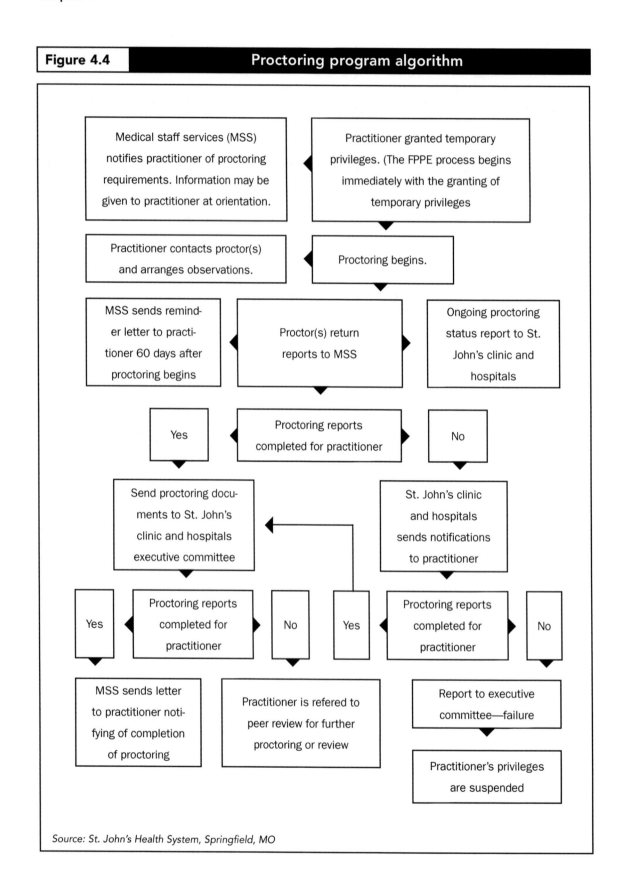

Source: St. John's Health System, Springfield, MO

Figure 4.5	Proctoring letter and checklist

> **Note:** *Upon granting privileges, the officers of the clinic and hospitals are notified of the responsibility to evaluate the care of the practitioner. It is also interesting to note on this document the communication of the expectation that this review is completed by the eighth week of practice.*

[Date]

Dear [*chairman of the section*]:

The St. John's Clinic executive committee and St. John's Hospital(s) executive committee(s) are responsible for proctoring and monitoring all new physicians. This letter is by way of instruction to you to assist us in this matter.

Dr. [*practitioner's name*] has recently started practicing at St. John's Clinic and St. John's Hospital(s), and we would like you to assist us in the proctoring process. Proctoring can be done by you or another member of your division whom you so designate. Please complete the attached checklist, including any operative notes or chart documentation, and submit it to St. John's Health System medical staff services for review by the clinic and hospital(s) executive committee(s). The documents may be forwarded via confidential fax [*fax number*]. Please note that the proctoring process is expected to be complete by the new physician's eighth week of service.

We are all responsible for the success of our new physicians and for ensuring quality of care for our patients. Thank you for your assistance in this process. If you have any questions, please contact us or St. John's Health System medical staff services at [*phone number*].

Sincerely,

_____   _____
President, St. John's Clinic   Chief of Staff, St. John's Hospital

cc: General Counsel
       Human Resources
       Medical Staff Services

Figure 4.5	Proctoring letter and checklist (cont.)

Proctoring program checklist

Name of physician: _____
(Please print)

Proctor: _____
(Please print)

Return date: _____
(Please print)

Completion date to be no later than eight weeks of service

Proctoring requirements:

Primary care:

- Monitor care of three to five patients, to include major and minor illness processes

- Provide summary of chart documentation, timely chart completion, and appropriate office charges per completion of proctor's report: medical/admission

Procedural based:

- Observe three to five surgical procedures, to include major and minor types (attach operative note)

- Provide summary of chart documentation, timely chart completion, and appropriate office charges per completion of proctor's report—surgical/procedural

Notice the two areas above where "appropriate office charges" are listed. Generally, focused professional practice evaluation (FPPE) would not encompass the appropriateness of office charges. However, in St. John's Health System, corporate compliance responsibilities dictate that charts are accurately diagnosed and thus coded for reimbursement from Medicare, Medicaid, and other third-party payers. Therefore, this aspect is included in the FPPE review.

Overall observations: _____

_____

Please submit all information to St. John's Health System Medical Staff Services

Source: St. John's Health System, Springfield, MO

Figure 4.6	Procedure log to document proctored cases or privilege maintenance

Note: *Most organizations have a fairly reliable method of identifying patients treated or procedures done by a particular physician. However, tracking the patients/procedures for advance practice professionals, such as nurse practitioners and physician assistants, is problematic in most organizations. To overcome this challenge, St. John's Health System instructs the individual nurse practitioner or physician assistant to provide a list of patients to whom they have provided care. Further, the supervising/collaborating physician is asked to attest to the accuracy of the list. This list is then used to identify charts for review.*

Practitioner name: _____

Procedure: _____

	Date	Medical record #	Comments
1.			
2.			
3.			
4.			
5.			
6.			
7.			
8.			
9.			
10.			
11.			
12.			

_____
Supervising/collaborating physician signature/date

_____
Supervising/collaborating physician printed name

Source: St. John's Health System, Springfield, MO

Editor's note

St. John's Health System developed a simplified method of outlining and recording the progress of the FPPE process through the Springfield and regional hospitals, as well as through the clinic. As mentioned in the profile at the beginning of this chapter, because St. John's is a very integrated system, the organization recognizes its responsibility to evaluate care provided in all settings. Therefore, the forms included in this book begin with a selection of diagnoses to be evaluated at the clinic level.

St. John's has a site-specific criteria-based core privileging system throughout the network. The organization determined that, for primary care specialists in general, at least three to five charts will be reviewed retrospectively, and for procedural-based specialists, three to five surgical procedures will be observed. To outline the specifics of the expectations, each section has developed or are in the process of developing a very simple FPPE form.

On each form (Figures 4.7-4.13) there is a section for chart review. The specific charts are selected based upon the scope of the privileges granted. The proctor designates the diagnoses or procedures that he or she wishes to evaluate (which reflect the new applicant's privileges). These charts reflect high-volume, high-risk, and/or problem prone-patients. In addition to this obligation, the specialties have also designated certain diagnoses and/or procedures where concurrent proctoring is required.

Figure 4.7	Cardiovascular proctor checklist

> **Note:** *This specialty has further separated the focused professional practice evaluation expectations into invasive, noninvasive, and electrophysiology. For further explaination, see editor's note on p. 88.*

Cardiovascular disease: Invasive

St. John's Clinic

- ❏ Clinic chart review #1 (pacemaker management—electrophysiology physicians)
- ❏ Clinic chart review #2 (congestive heart failure)
- ❏ Clinic chart review #3 (coronary disease #1)
- ❏ Clinic chart review #4 (coronary disease #2)

St. John's Hospital—Springfield

- ❏ Chart review
- ❏ Chart review
- ❏ Chart review
- ❏ Chart review

Two or more of the following procedures are required to be proctored:

- ❏ Percutaneous transluminal coronary angioplasty/percutaneous coronary intervention/stent—percutaneous coronary intervention
- ❏ Diagnostic cardiac catheterization
- ❏ Intracoronary stents

Cardiovascular disease: Noninvasive

St. John's Clinic

- ❏ Stress echocardiography—exercise
- ❏ Stress echocardiography—pharmacologic
- ❏ EKG interpretation
- ❏ Nuclear stress
- ❏ Clinic chart review #1 (coronary disease)
- ❏ Clinic chart review #2 (valvular heart diseases)

St. John's Hospital—Springfield

- ❏ Chart review
- ❏ Chart review
- ❏ Chart review
- ❏ Chart review

Figure 4.7	Cardiovascular proctor checklist (cont.)

Two or more of the following procedures are required to be proctored:

- ❑ Stress echocardiography—exercise
- ❑ Stress echocardiography—pharmacologic
- ❑ EKG interpretation
- ❑ 2D echocardiography

St. John's Hospital—Springfield: Electrophysiology physicians

Two or more of the following procedures are required to be proctored:

- ❑ Pacemaker insertion
- ❑ Automatic implantable cardioverter defibrillator
- ❑ Holter monitor interpretation
- ❑ EKG interpretation
- ❑ Electrophysiology study
- ❑ Catheter ablation:
  - o Supraventricular tachycardia
  - o Atrial fibrillation/pulmonary vein isolation

St. John's regional hospitals

- ❑ Over read #1
- ❑ Over read #2
- ❑ Over read #3
- ❑ Over read #4
- ❑ Over read #5

St. John's Clinic chart reviews may meet the above proctoring requirements by following the patient from initial clinic visit, inpatient care, and postop clinic visit for a single diagnosis.

Source: St. John's Health System, Springfield, MO

Figure 4.8	Cardiovascular and thoracic surgery proctor checklist

Note: *For further explaination, see editor's note on p. 88.*

St. John's Clinic

- ❏ Clinic chart review #1 (disease of lung)
- ❏ Clinic chart review #2 (valve disease)
- ❏ Clinic chart review #3 (coronary disease #1)
- ❏ Clinic chart review #4 (coronary disease #2)
- ❏ Clinic chart review #5 (vascular disease and treatment)

St. John's Hospital—Springfield

- ❏ Chart review
- ❏ Chart review

Two or more of the following procedures are required to be proctored:

- ❏ Coronary artery bypass graft—on and off pump
- ❏ Valve procedure
- ❏ Intraoperative infection control procedures
- ❏ Ventilator management
- ❏ Thoracotomy
- ❏ Open vascular procedures
- ❏ Endovascular procedures

Cardio vascular and thoracic surgery noninvasive vascular laboratory studies interpretation

St. John's regional hospitals

- ❏ Over read #1
- ❏ Over read #2
- ❏ Over read #3
- ❏ Over read #4
- ❏ Over read #5

St. John's Clinic chart reviews may meet the above proctoring requirements by following the patient from initial clinic visit, inpatient care, and postop clinic visit for a single diagnosis.

Source: St. John's Health System, Springfield, MO

Figure 4.9	Emergency medicine proctor checklist

Note: *For further explaination, see editor's note on p. 88.*

St. John's Hospitals—Springfield and regional

❑ Chart review
❑ Chart review
❑ Chart review
❑ Chart review
❑ Chart review

Three or more of the following procedures are required to be proctored:

❑ Abdominal pain management
❑ Chest pain management
❑ Pneumonia management
❑ Trauma management
❑ Orthopedic management of fractures/dislocations
❑ Stroke management
❑ Cardiopulmonary resuscitation management
❑ Central line placement
❑ Lumbar puncture
❑ Congestive heart failure management
❑ Procedural sedation and analgesia
❑ Respiratory distress/failure management
❑ Laceration management
❑ Rapid sequence intubation

Emergency medicine, emergency trauma center acute care center

St. John's Hospital—Springfield

❑ Burn management
❑ Removal of foreign bodies
❑ Slitlamp for ocular exam
❑ Injection of bursa or joint
❑ Application of splint and plaster molds

Source: St. John's Health System, Springfield, MO

Figure 4.10	Family medicine/sports medicine proctor checklist

Note: For further explaination, see editor's note on p. 88.

St. John's Clinic

Two or more of the following procedures are required to be proctored:

❑ Cast application
❑ Injection of tendon, ligament, joint
❑ Joint fracture reduction under local anesthesia
❑ Interpretation of routine radiographic study
❑ Shoulder dislocation, anterior, uncomplicated

Family medicine without obstetrics

St. John's Clinic

❑ Clinic chart review
❑ Clinic chart review
❑ Clinic chart review
❑ Clinic chart review
❑ Clinic chart review

St. John's Hospital—Springfield

❑ Chart review
❑ Chart review
❑ Chart review
❑ Chart review
❑ Chart review

Two or more of the following are required to be proctored:

> Note that not all concurrent proctoring is procedural. In these instances, the organization is expecting the proctor to evaluate the care as it is being given.

❑ Code management
❑ Pneumonia management
❑ Gastrointestinal (GI) infection
❑ Urinary tract infection
❑ Pediatric management

| Figure 4.10 | Family medicine/sports medicine proctor checklist (cont.) |

St. John's Regional Hospitals

- ❑ Chart review
- ❑ Chart review
- ❑ Chart review
- ❑ Chart review
- ❑ Chart review

Two or more of the following procedures are required to be proctored:

- ❑ Code management
- ❑ Pneumonia management
- ❑ GI infection
- ❑ Exercise stress testing
- ❑ Ventilator management

Family medicine with obstetrics

St. John's Clinic

- ❑ Clinic chart review
- ❑ Clinic chart review
- ❑ Clinic chart review
- ❑ Clinic chart review
- ❑ Clinic chart review

Two or more of the following procedures are required to be proctored:

- ❑ Obstetrics management (required)
- ❑ History and physical
- ❑ Flexible proctosigmoidoscopy (if applicable)
- ❑ Vasectomy (if applicable)
- ❑ EKG interpretation

Family medicine with obstetrics and gynecology

St. John's Regional Hospitals: Aurora and Berryville

- ❑ Chart review
- ❑ Chart review
- ❑ Chart review
- ❑ Chart review
- ❑ Chart review

| Figure 4.10 | Family medicine/sports medicine proctor checklist (cont.) |

Two or more of the following procedures are required to be proctored:

- ❏ C-section
- ❏ Delivery of twins, vaginal, including normal and breech second delivery
- ❏ Repair of 4° laceration
- ❏ Ventilator management
- ❏ Amniocentesis

Family medicine with gastroenterology

St. John's Regional Hospitals

- ❏ Chart review
- ❏ Chart review
- ❏ Chart review
- ❏ Chart review
- ❏ Chart review

Two or more of the following procedures are required to be proctored:

- ❏ Esophagogastroduodenoscopy: Cassville and St. Francis
- ❏ Colonoscopy: Aurora, Cassville, and St. Francis
- ❏ Code management
- ❏ Pneumonia management
- ❏ Ventilator management

Family medicine with newborn

St. John's Regional Hospitals: Aurora, Berryville, Lebanon

- ❏ Chart review
- ❏ Chart review
- ❏ Chart review
- ❏ Chart review
- ❏ Chart review

Two or more of the following procedures are required to be proctored:

- ❏ Circumcision
- ❏ Venipuncture
- ❏ Arterial blood gases
- ❏ Central and arterial line placement
- ❏ Lumbar puncture

Source: St. John's Health System, Springfield, MO

Figure 4.11	Gastroenterology proctor checklist

> **Note:** *For further explaination, see editor's note on p. 88.*

St. John's Clinic

- ❑ Consultation #1
- ❑ Consultation #2
- ❑ Consultation #3
- ❑ Consultation #4
- ❑ Consultation #5
- ❑ Clinic chart review #1 (chronic liver disease)
- ❑ Clinic chart review #2 (gastrointestinal [GI] bleed)
- ❑ Clinic chart review #3 (abdominal pain)
- ❑ Clinic chart review #4 (inflammatory bowel)

St. John's Hospital—Springfield

- ❑ Upper GI therapeutic procedure #1
- ❑ Upper GI therapeutic procedure #2
- ❑ Lower GI therapeutic procedure #1
- ❑ Lower GI therapeutic procedure #2
- ❑ Percutaneous endoscopic gastronomy (PEG) or endoscopic retrograde cholangiopancreatogram (ERCP)

St. John's Clinic chart reviews may meet the above proctoring requirements by following the patient from initial clinic visit, inpatient care, and postop clinic visit for a single diagnosis.

Source: St. John's Health System, Springfield, MO

Figure 4.12	Neurological surgery proctor checklist

Note: *For further explaination, see editor's note on p. 88.*

St. John's Clinic

- ❏ Clinic chart review #1 (craniotomy)
- ❏ Clinic chart review #2 (laminectomy)
- ❏ Clinic chart review #3 (ventricular shunt)
- ❏ Clinic chart review #4 (cervical fusion)
- ❏ Clinic chart review #5 (spinal cord surgery)

St. John's Hospital—Springfield

- ❏ Chart review
- ❏ Chart review
- ❏ Chart review
- ❏ Chart review
- ❏ Chart review

Two or more of the following procedures are required to be proctored:

- ❏ Craniotomy
- ❏ Laminectomy
- ❏ Ventricular shunt
- ❏ Cervical fusion
- ❏ Craniotomy with deep brain stimulators

Neurological surgery, neuroendovascular

St. John's Clinic

- ❏ Clinic chart review #1 (craniotomy)
- ❏ Clinic chart review #2 (laminectomy)
- ❏ Clinic chart review #3 (cranial or spinal vascular malformation)
- ❏ Clinic chart review #4 (cerebral aneurysm)
- ❏ Clinic chart review #5 (spinal cord surgery)

St. John's Hospital—Springfield

- ❏ Chart review
- ❏ Chart review
- ❏ Chart review
- ❏ Chart review

Figure 4.12	Neurological surgery proctor checklist (cont.)

Two or more of the following procedures are required to be proctored:

- ❏ Coil occlusion of aneurysms
- ❏ Combined carotid arteriography and carotid artery stenting (if granted this privilege)
- ❏ Endovascular embolization of vascular malformations
- ❏ Acute stroke therapy

Neurological surgery pediatric

St. John's Clinic

- ❏ Clinic chart review #1 (cranial surgery)
- ❏ Clinic chart review #2 (spinal surgery)
- ❏ Clinic chart review #3 (congenital central nervous system [CNS] surgery)
- ❏ Clinic chart review #4 (pediatric epilepsy surgery)

St. John's Hospital—Springfield

- ❏ Chart review
- ❏ Chart review
- ❏ Chart review
- ❏ Chart review
- ❏ Chart review

Two or more of the following procedures are required to be proctored:

- ❏ Pediatric epilepsy surgery
- ❏ Spinal surgery
- ❏ Pediatric neurosurgical repair of congenital CNS anomalies
- ❏ Cranial surgery

St. John's Clinic chart reviews may meet the above proctoring requirements by following the patient from initial clinic visit, inpatient care, and postop clinic visit for a single diagnosis.

Source: St. John's Health System, Springfield, MO

Figure 4.13	Urology proctor checklist

Note: For further explaination, see editor's note on p. 88.

St. John's Clinic
- ❏ Clinic chart review #1 (prostate cancer)
- ❏ Clinic chart review #2 (urinary incontinence)
- ❏ Cystourethroscopy
- ❏ Biopsy of prostate
- ❏ Vasectomy

St. John's Hospital—Springfield and St. John's Regional Hospitals—Aurora, Berryville, and St. Francis

- ❏ Chart review
- ❏ Chart review
- ❏ Chart review
- ❏ Chart review
- ❏ Chart review

Two or more of the following procedures are required to be proctored:

- ❏ Major bladder procedure
- ❏ Transurethral prostatectomy
- ❏ Major male pelvic procedure
- ❏ Laparoscopic nephrectomy
- ❏ Urinary incontinence procedure

St. John's Clinic chart reviews may meet the above proctoring requirements by following the patient from initial clinic visit, inpatient care, and postop clinic visit for a single diagnosis.

Source: St. John's Health System, Springfield, MO

XYZ Medical Center

Note: *XYZ Medical Center is not the actual name of this organization. The organization wishes to remain anonymous as a contributor to this book.*

XYZ Medical Center has a medical staff featuring 200 licensed independent practitioners and consultants. The Joint Commission (formerly JCAHO)–accredited organization is in an urban location and has 46 hospital beds and 38 rehabilitation-oriented nursing home beds. In addition, it has a mobile clinic outfitted with two exam rooms that serves patients in rural areas, as well as partnerships with several other healthcare organizations in the same region with which it shares resources.

The medical staff coordinator for XYZ Medical Center initiated the organization's focused professional practice evaluation (FPPE) development process by independently researching FPPE and exchanging information with her peers. Then the medical staff coordinator passed this information on to the chief of medicine, who developed the new FPPE forms.

XYZ Medical Center created its professional practice evaluation form for a number of clinical services based on the six areas of general competencies, which were developed through the efforts of the Accreditation Council for Graduate Medical Education and the American Board of Medical Specialties. The medical services form (used to evaluate all practitioners, including physicians, advanced practice nurses, and physician assistants) and the dental services form are included in this chapter.

Initially, the medical center developed these forms to evaluate newly privileged practitioners and to meet The Joint Commission's focused professional practice requirement. However, the medical center intends to broaden the use of these forms to evaluate all practitioners. Based on this new intent, a random selection of each practitioner's patient charts will be evaluated using these criteria. The assessment will simply be another component of the current ongoing professional practice evaluation.

Figure 5.1	Medicine service professional practice evaluation

Provider: _____

Specialty: _____

This would denote the time frame of review—for example, first or second month of appointment.

Evaluation period: _____

Review type:
- ❑ Focused review at initial appointment
- ❑ Biannual review, random selection of charts
- ❑ Focused review for assessment of ability to deliver safe, high-quality patient care
  Chart selected because: Clinical indicator not met: [indicator listed]
  or [other reason listed]

Factor	Evaluation criteria	Evaluation (* requires further comment on last page)
Patient care: Provides care that is compassionate, appropriate, and effective for the promotion of health, prevention of illness, treatment of disease, and supportive at the end of life	❑ Meets customer service expectations (review of staff and patient compliments and complaints) ❑ Refrains from use of disallowed abbreviations (chart review) ❑ Complies with medication reconciliation policy (chart review) ❑ Addresses active medical problems in a timely fashion (list charts reviewed) ❑ Practices within scope of granted privileges (list charts reviewed) ❑ Demonstrated current competency in the privileges requested (list charts reviewed)	❑ Satisfactory ❑ Unsatisfactory* Comments: _____ _____ _____ _____
Medical/clinical knowledge: Demonstrates knowledge of established and evolving biomedical, clinical, and social sciences and applies this knowledge to patient care and the education of others	❑ Maintains board certification (if board certified) ❑ Meets faculty continuing medical education requirements ❑ Participates in resident/student teaching ❑ Serves as a sponsoring physician for a physician assistant ❑ Serves as an advanced cardiac life supprt/basic cardiac life support instructor ❑ Presented a medical education lecture during this rating period (not required) ❑ Demonstrated current competency in the privileges requested (list charts reviewed)	❑ Satisfactory ❑ Unsatisfactory* Comments: _____ _____ _____ _____

Factor	Data source	Evaluation (* requires further comment on last page)
Practice-based learning and improvement: Uses specific evidence and methods to investigate, evaluate, and improve patient care practices	❑ Participates in preprocedure timeouts ❑ N/A due to scope of practice ❑ Participates in performance or process-improvement task forces, workgroups, or committees as requested ❑ Remains abreast of medical advances in his or her area of expertise and incorporates this information to deliver care that meets contemporary standards of care (chart review)	❑ Satisfactory ❑ Unsatisfactory* Comments: _____ _____ _____ _____

| Figure 5.1 | Medicine service professional practice evaluation (cont.) |

Factor	Data source	Evaluation
Interpersonal and communication skills: Demonstrates interpersonal and communication skills that enables him or her to establish and maintain professional relationships with patients, families, and other members of health-care teams	❑ Authors clinical encounter notes that are free of significant documentation deficiencies with regard to (chart review): • Pertinent history and review of systems • Pertinent physical exam • Relevant assessment and plan ❑ Electronic medical records entries are appropriate in tone and content (chart review) ❑ Provides adequate patient information when requesting specialist consultations • Indication for consultant is clear • Pertinent clinical data is provided ❑ Provides appropriate consultative evaluation, treatment, and follow-up recommendations (chart review) ❑ Meets customer service expectations (review of staff and patient complaints)	❑ Satisfactory ❑ Unsatisfactory* Comments: _____ _____ _____ _____

Factor	**Data source** (* requires further comment on last page)	**Evaluation** (* requires further comment on last page)

Professionalism: Demonstrates behaviors that reflect a commitment to continuous professional development, ethical practice, understanding and sensitivity to diversity, and a respectable attitude toward patients, the medical profession, and society	❑ Participates in peer review as requested
	    ❑ N/A during this rating period
	❑ Participates on committees as requested
	    ❑ N/A during this rating period
	❑ Absence of validated disruptive or unprofessional behavior
	
	Staff meeting attendance:
	attended [*insert number*] of [*insert number*] meetings
	
	Observed behavior suggestive of possible chemical dependency: ❑ No ❑ Yes*
		❑ Satisfactory
		❑ Unsatisfactory*
		
		Comments: _____
		_____
		_____
		_____

Systems-based practice: Understands the contexts and systems in which healthcare is provided and applies this knowledge to improve and optimize healthcare	Complies with safety, security, and privacy policies (ongoing monitoring) ❑ Usually ❑ Sometimes ❑ Rarely Arrives to work on time (supervisor/team leader evaluation) ❑ Usually ❑ Sometimes ❑ Rarely Arranges proper clinical coverage during planned absences (supervisor/team leader evaluation) ❑ Usually ❑ Sometimes ❑ Rarely Complies with hand-off communication policy (supervisor evaluation)	❑ Satisfactory ❑ Unsatisfactory* Comments: _____ _____ _____ _____

Evaluator's comments: _____

Evaluation completed by (supervisor's name and date): _____

This position is equivalent to a specialty or subspecialty director within the department of medicine.

Chief of medicine's comments: _____

Chief of medicine's signature and date: _____

Source: XYZ Medical Center

Figure 5.2	Dental service professional practice evaluation

Note: *Using the medicine service professional practice evaluation form as a template, the dentistry service adapted the content for the practice of dentistry.*

Provider: _____

> This would denote the time frame of review—for example, first or second month of appointment.

Evaluation period: _____

Review type: ❑ Focused review at initial appointment
❑ Biannual review, random selection of charts
❑ Focused review for assessment of ability to deliver safe, high-quality patient care
   Chart selected because: Clinical indicator not met _____ (indicator listed)
   _____ or _____ (other reason listed) _____

Factor	Evaluation criteria	Evaluation (* requires further comment on last page)
Patient care: Provides care that is compassionate, appropriate, and effective for the promotion of dental health, prevention of dental disease, and treatment of dental disease	❑ Meets customer service expectations (review of staff and patient compliments and complaints) ❑ Refrains from use of disallowed abbreviations (chart review) ❑ Complies with medication reconciliation policy (chart review) ❑ Addresses active medical problems in a timely fashion (list charts reviewed) ❑ Practices within scope of granted privileges (list charts reviewed) ❑ Demonstrated current competency in the privileges requested (list charts reviewed)	❑ Satisfactory ❑ Unsatisfactory* Comments: _____ _____ _____ _____
Dental/medical/ clinical knowledge: Demonstrates knowledge of established and evolving biomedical, clinical and social sciences, and applies this knowledge to patient care and the education of others	❑ Meets facility continuing medical education requirements ❑ Participates in dental hygiene student training	❑ Satisfactory ❑ Unsatisfactory* Comments: _____ _____ _____ _____

Figure 5.2	Dental service professional practice evaluation (cont.)

Factor	Data source	Evaluation (* requires further comment on last page)
Practice-based learning and improvement: Uses specific evidence and methods to investigate, evaluate, and improve patient care practices	❑ Participates in preprocedure timeouts ❑ Participates in performance or process-improvement task forces, workgroups, or committees, as requested ❑ Remains abreast of medical advances in dentistry and incorporates this information to deliver care that meets contemporary standards of care (chart review)	❑ Satisfactory ❑ Unsatisfactory* Comments: _____ _____ _____
Interpersonal and communication skills: Demonstrates interpersonal and communication skills that enables him or her to establish and maintain professional relationships with patients, families, and other members of healthcare teams	❑ Authors clinical encounter notes that are free of significant documentation deficiencies with regard to (chart review): • Pertinent medical history • Pertinent dental exam • Relevant assessment and plan ❑ Electronic patient records entries are appropriate in tone and content (chart review) ❑ Provides adequate patient information when requesting specialist consultations • Indication for consultant is clear • Pertinent clinical data is provided ❑ Provides appropriate consultative evaluation, treatment, and follow-up recommendations (chart review) ❑ Meets customer service expectations (review of staff and patient complaints)	❑ Satisfactory ❑ Unsatisfactory* Comments: _____ _____ _____ _____

Factor	Data source (* requires further comment on last page)	Evaluation (* requires further comment on last page)
Professionalism: Demonstrates behaviors that reflect a commitment to continuous professional development, ethical practice, understanding and sensitivity to diversity, and a respectable attitude toward patients, the dental profession, and society	❑ Participates in peer review as requested ❑ N/A during this rating period ❑ Absence of validated disruptive or unprofessional behavior Staff meeting attendance: attended [insert number] of [insert number] meetings Observed behavior suggestive of possible chemical dependency: ❑ No ❑ Yes*	❑ Satisfactory ❑ Unsatisfactory* Comments: _____ _____ _____ _____
Systems-based practice: Understands the contexts and systems in which healthcare is provided and applies this knowledge to improve and optimize healthcare	Complies with safety, security, and privacy policies (ongoing monitoring) ❑ Usually ❑ Sometimes ❑ Rarely Arrives to work on time ❑ Usually ❑ Sometimes ❑ Rarely Arranges proper clinical coverage during planned absences ❑ Usually ❑ Sometimes ❑ Rarely Complies with hand-off communication policy (supervisor evaluation)	❑ Satisfactory ❑ Unsatisfactory* Comments: _____ _____ _____ _____

Evaluator's comments: _____

Evaluation completed by: (clinician's name and date): _____

Chief of of dentistry's comments: _____

Chief of of dentistry's signature and date: _____

Source: XYZ Medical Center

Additional FPPE documents

The authors included the following documents because they exhibit exemplary focused professional practice evaluation practices.

Please refer to the notes on the individual forms for additional explanations.

Figure 6.1	Focused professional practice evaluation process

Note: *This outline shows the similarities and differences between focused professional practice evaluation (FPPE) for new applicants or for a current applicant requesting new privileges, and FPPE for existing practitioners whose performance has raised questions. According to this organization's process, the final report is placed in the practitioner's credentials file.*

Triggers for FPPE

Practitioner has credentials to suggest competence	Questions arise regarding practitioner's practice
Initially requested privileges (at initial appointment or new for current appointee)	Referral from risk management
	Occurrence screen
Reentry (whether or not mandated by state medical board)	Outlier from OPPE
	Clinical practice trend
Low- or no-volume practitioner	Single incident
	Failed collegial intervention
	Failed action plan
Credentials Committee	QA Committee

Alternate outcomes

Step 1: Select FPPE monitoring method

Prospective proctoring	Concurrent proctoring	Retrospective proctoring
Chart review		Case review
Interview others	Simulation	External peer review
Monitoring patterns		Other

Step 2: Develop action plan for the practitioner

Alternate Step 2:

Require practitioner to complete additional educational activities
Concurrent consultation
Proctoring (prospective, concurrent, retrospective)
Coadmitting privileges
Other

Recommend investigation of practitioner

Step 3:

Develop performance improvement plan for the hospital

| Figure 6.1 | Focused professional practice evaluation process (cont.) |

Note: *The preceeding outline was based on the following Joint Commission (formerly JCAHO) elements of performance (EP) from standard MS.4.30:*

Triggers

EP1: A period of FPPE is implemented for all initially requested privileges

EP5: The triggers that indicate the need for performance monitoring are clearly defined

EP6: The decision to assign a period of performance monitoring to further assess current clinical competence, practice behavior, and ability to perform the requested privilege

FPPE process alternatives

EP2: The organized medical staff develops criteria to be used for evaluating the performance of practitioners when issues affecting the provision of safe, high-quality patient care are identified

EP3: The performance monitoring process is clearly defined and includes each of the following elements:
- Criteria for conducting performance monitoring
- Method for establishing a monitoring plan specific to the requested privilege
- Method for determining the duration of performance monitoring
- Circumstances under which monitoring by an external source is required

EP7: Criteria are developed that determine the type of monitoring to be conducted

EP8: The measures employed to resolve performance issues are clearly defined

FPPE process implementation

EP4: FPPE is consistently implemented in accordance with the criteria and requirements defined by the organized medical staff

EP9: The measures employed to resolve performance issues are consistently implemented

Source: Carolinas Healthcare System, Charlotte, NC.

| Figure 6.2 | Guide to drafting a focused professional practice evaluation policy |

Recommended elements of a focused professional practice evaluation (FPPE) policy:

- Purpose
- Medical staff oversight
- Ethical positions of the medical staff
- Scope of proctoring program
- Responsibilities
- Methods
- Procedure
- Reporting: Results and recommendations

I. Purpose

The policy should state the reasons for conducting FPPE and explain its place in the organizational scheme. Although the policy may or may not specifically reference The Joint Commission standards, the reasons for conducting FPPE should extend beyond the goal of meeting regulatory compliance. The primary goal should be to use FPPE as another tool to assess and ensure competence as part of the organization's ongoing commitment to quality.

II. Medical staff oversight

1. Identify which individuals or group(s) in the medical staff (e.g., the credentials committee, department chairs, the medical executive committee, or other) will have primary oversight of the FPPE process.

2. Discuss how the FPPE process will be integrated with the organization's ongoing professional practice evaluation (OPPE) process and the clinical privileging system.

III. Ethical positions of the medical staff

The FPPE policy should address the following ethical concerns:

- Conflicts of interest
- Disclosure to patients
- Consent issues
- Intervention by the proctor
- Indemnification for proctors

IV. Scope of the proctoring program

The policy should define proctoring and delineate the activities that comprise it—including whether the organization will use the term proctoring interchangeably with FPPE. (The Greeley Company generally recommends that the terms proctoring and FPPE be used interchangeably.) In addition, the policy should define the methods to be employed and the individuals to whom the program applies (e.g., initial applicants, currently privileged individuals requesting additional privileges).

V. Responsibilities

The policy should answer the following questions:

| Figure 6.2 | Guide to drafting a focused professional practice evaluation policy (cont.) |

- Who will create the practitioner-specific FPPE plan?
- Who will assign proctors?
- Who will collect the data?
- Who will analyze the data and make recommendations?

The policy should clearly delineate the duties of the proctoree, proctors, department chairs, credentials committee, medical executive committee, and the medical staff services and quality departments.

VI. Methods
Typically, some or all of the following methods are used in an FPPE program:

- Prospective proctoring
- Concurrent proctoring (i.e., real-time proctoring)
- Retrospective proctoring
- Teleproctoring
- Crossover proctoring (i.e., proctoring of clinical work is done at another institution, but a proctor from your organization is used)
- Anticipatory proctoring (i.e., proctoring is accomplished before the applicant exercises privileges on site; with this advance proctoring, the on-site FPPE may be reduced)
- Simulation

The policy should also outline the circumstances for proctoring from an external source.

VII. Procedure
This section of the FPPE policy provides guidelines for addressing logistical challenges:

- Data: What should be collected, how should it be collected, and how much of it should be collected?
- Scheduling: How can proctoring be scheduled efficiently?
- Are substitute proctors allowed?

VIII. Reporting
The FPPE policy should address how and when the data that has been gathered and analyzed will be reported—including the method for making recommendations. Most often the endpoint is reached when competency is established, thus ending FPPE and triggering the start of the routine OPPE monitoring process.

Source: The Greenley Company, a division of HCPro, Inc., Marblehead, MA.

Figure 6.3	Sample focused professional practice evaluation plan for a newly trained and board-certified cardiologist

Skill being evaluated	Activity being evaluated	Method for evaluating activity
Cognitive skills	10 cases of varied diagnoses, including myocardial infarction, congestive heart failure, etc. (covering privileges granted)	Retrospective review
Procedural skills	2 diagnostic and 4 interventional catheterizations	Concurrent proctoring

Projected time frame: within 90 days of being granted clinical privileges.

Source: The Greeley Company, a division of HCPro, Inc., Marblehead, MA.

Figure 6.4	Sample focused professional practice evaluation for a nurse midwife

Note: *Delineating the focused professional practice evaluation (FPPE) process and components is a detailed process. However, the outcome (an FPPE plan for a particular practitioner) should be clear, concise, and communicated to all involved parties. This sample FPPE for a nurse midwife models those parameters. This document would then be provided the applicant, the medical staff office, the quality improvement department, and nursing units as applicable (in this case, labor and delivery and the nursery).*

Skill being evaluated	Activity being evaluated	Method for evaluating activity
Cognitive skills	Manage midwifery elements of (n) moderate-risk cases after consultation with physician	Retrospective review
	Manage midwifery elements of (n) high-risk cases after consultation with physician	Prospective review
Procedural skills	Deliver (n) patients and manage (n) infants at delivery	Concurrent proctoring
	Perform (n) amniotomy procedures	Concurrent proctoring
	Perform (n) episiotomy and repair procedures	Concurrent proctoring
	Perform (n) vacuum extractions	Concurrent proctoring

Projected time frame: within 90 days of being granted clinical privileges.

Source: The Greeley Company, a division of HCPro, Inc., Marblehead, MA.

Follow these simple steps to earn your CE credits

Dear reader,

We are pleased to be able to help you achieve continuing education credits through *The FPPE Toolbox: Field-Tested Documents for Credentialing, Competency, and Compliance*. This section will tell you, in simple steps, how to take the quiz and earn the CE credits. However, please feel free to contact Customer Service at 800/650-6787, 781/639-1872 or e-mail *customerservice@hcpro.com* with any questions.

Note: *The FPPE Toolbox: Field-Tested Documents for Credentialing, Competency, and Compliance*, has been approved by the National Association Medical Staff Services for up to six continuing education credits. Accreditation of this educational program in no way implies endorsement or sponsorship by NAMSS.

To earn your NAMMS credits, simply contact HCPro, Inc., within one year of receiving this book and we will provide you with your username and password. Then log-in, take the exam, and score at least 70%. Once you pass the exam, you can print out your certificate! For a detailed explanation of each step, see below.

Instructions to access and take the online quiz:

I. Gaining access to *www.hcprofessor.com* and the online quiz

1. Call Customer Service at 800/650-6787 or 781/639-1872. Let them know you are calling to get access for *The FPPE Toolbox: Field-Tested Documents for Credentialing, Competency, and Compliance* book quiz.

2. State order code: FPPEQZ

3. Customer Service will provide you with a username and password via e-mail within 48 hours. These enable you to log on to the HCProfessor Web site and take the online quiz to earn your CE credits.

II. Logging onto the Web site and accessing the quiz

1. Go to *www.hcprofessor.com*.

2. Click on the Log On command in the left hand navigation column.

3. Log on using your access, which you received from Customer Service (the username and password).

4. Once logged on, you will see the online quiz for *The FPPE Toolbox: Field-Tested Documents for Credentialing, Competency, and Compliance*.

5. Upon completion of the test, click on "submit."

If you have any questions about using the Web site or accessing the quiz, please call HCPro, Inc. at 888/209-7182. You may also e-mail us at *HCProfessortechsupport@hcpro.com*.

III. Earning the CE credits

You have up to one year after receipt of this book to complete the exam, and a passing grade of 70% is required for the certification of your continuing education hours completed with this activity. Your passing grade will then allow you access online to a certificate of completion. The exam grading and access to the certificate is immediate. If you fail the exam on your first try, you will be allowed to retake the exam as many times as necessary within a 30-day access period.